Fifty Cases in Dermatological Medicine

Daniel Creamer

Department of Dermatology
King's College Hospital
Denmark Hill
London SE5 9RS

Anthony du Vivier

Department of Dermatology
King's College Hospital
Denmark Hill
London SE5 9RS

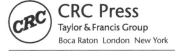

CRC Press
Taylor & Francis Group
Boca Raton London New York

CRC Press is an imprint of the
Taylor & Francis Group, an **informa** business

A TAYLOR & FRANCIS BOOK

CRC Press
Taylor & Francis Group
6000 Broken Sound Parkway NW, Suite 300
Boca Raton, FL 33487-2742

First issued in paperback 2019

© 2005 by Taylor & Francis Group, LLC
CRC Press is an imprint of Taylor & Francis Group, an Informa business

No claim to original U.S. Government works

ISBN-13: 978-1-84184-143-4 (hbk)
ISBN-13: 978-0-367-39344-1 (pbk)

Visit the Taylor & Francis Web site at
http://www.taylorandfrancis.com

and the CRC Press Web site at
http://www.crcpress.com

Dedication

This book is dedicated to our wives, Katherine and Judith.

Contents

vi   Contents

Preface

It is one of the joys of clinical dermatology that the interpretation of physical signs in the skin may provide the diagnosis to a systemic disease. Furthermore, the dermatologist must recognize that certain primary skin disorders may have important associations with internal pathology. The relationship between cutaneous and general medicine is the subject of this book of cases seen in the dermatology department at King's College Hospital, London.

We have aimed the material primarily at dermatologists in training, consultant dermatologists engaged in continuing professional development and candidates preparing for higher examinations in internal medicine and dermatology. *Fifty Cases in Dermatological Medicine* should also appeal to the general physician or general practitioner who is interested in dermatology.

A greater understanding of a disease and its management is often achieved through the study of an individual patient rather than a textbook. It is our hope that the 50 cases presented here exemplify this principle and stimulate further interest in dermatological medicine.

Acknowledgements

At King's College Hospital we are lucky to have a superlative department of medical photography and we would like to thank Yvonne Bartlett, David Langdon, Barry Pike, Lucy Wallace and Alex Dionysiou who have so skillfully recorded the clinical features presented in this book. Our special thanks go to Yvonne who has also carefully selected and prepared the images for publication.

We are grateful to current and previous members of the department of dermatology at King's College Hospital who have suggested cases for this book and have assisted in the preparation of the text. These contributors are cited in the list of contents. Since the patients were all jointly managed with colleagues in other departments at King's College Hospital we would like to acknowledge with gratitude our clinical collaborators: Dr F Calman, Professor L Cardoza, Dr C Clough, Dr J Costello, Sister Judy Davids, Mr J Desai, Dr S Devereux, Professor P Easterbrook, Dr M Edmonds, Dr I Forgacs, Dr B Gray, Dr S Hannam, Dr D Hutchinson, Mr A Leather, Professor A MacGregor, Dr W Marshall, Professor G Mufti, Dr A Pagliuca, Professor T Peters, Mr Porteous, Mr J Rennie, Mr J Roberts, Mr D Ross, Dr G Ruiz, Mr D Scott-Coombes, Dr A Stephens, Dr B Toone, Dr R Weeks, Professor R Williams.

Some of the patients were also seen by specialists in other hospitals and we would like to thank the following for their help: Dr E Baker, Professor C Black, Professor M Black, Dr A Bryceson, Dr D Lockwood, Dr M Moore, Professor M Pope, Dr S Qureshi, Dr R Russell-Jones, Dr F Vega-Lopez.

We would like to thank the St John's Institute of Dermatology for permission to reproduce the images used in figures 13a, 21b–c and 40c. A number of the cases have already been published in the dermatological literature and we would like to thank the publishers of the *British Journal of Dermatology, Clinical and Experimental Dermatology, Journal of the American Academy of Dermatology, Journal of the Royal Society of Medicine* and *Paediatric Dermatology*.

Finally, we would like to thank the patients presented in this book.

Abbreviations

ACE	angiotensin-converting enzyme	Hb	haemoglobin
ALP	alkaline phosphatase	H&E	haematoxylin and eosin
ANA	anti-nuclear antibody	IU	international unit
AST	aspartate transaminase	LFT	liver function test
ATLL	adult T-cell leukaemia-lymphoma	lymphs	lymphocytes
CD	cluster differentiation molecules	MCV	mean cell volume
CPK	creatinine phosphokinase	MRI	magnetic resonance imaging
CRP	C-reactive protein	MSU	midstream urine
CT	computed tomography	pANCA	anti-myeloperoxidase antibodies
ECG	electrocardiogram	PAS	periodic acid-Schiff
EMA	epithelial membrane antigen	plts	platelets
ENA	extractable nuclear antigen	PMN	polymorphonuclear cells
eos	eosinophils	RF	rheumatoid factor
ESR	erythrocyte sedimentation rate	TPHA	*Treponema pallidum*
FBC	full blood count		haemagglutinin assay
GGT	gamma-glutamyl transpeptidase	U&E	urea and electrolytes – and
GI	gastrointestinal		creatinine
GVHD	graft-versus-host disease	WCC	white cell count

Case 1
Haematemesis and warts

History

A 69-year-old man was admitted following an episode of haematemesis. For the previous 11 months he had suffered from dyspepsia, lethargy and night sweats. Latterly he had also noticed the development of numerous pruritic, warty papules on his trunk and limbs, and changes to the skin of the armpits, groins and neck.

Clinical findings

Cutaneous examination revealed myriads of small keratotic papules scattered over the trunk and limbs (Figures 1a, b). The axillary skin was hyperpigmented, thickened and thrown into coarse folds (Figure 1c). Similar velvety thickening was observed in the groins and at the nape of the neck. There were areas of papillomatosis at the commissures of the mouth (Figure 1d) and on the mucosa of the hard palate. The palms and soles were hyperkeratotic.

Examination of the abdomen demonstrated epigastric tenderness. There were palpable lymph nodes in the left supraclavicular fossa.

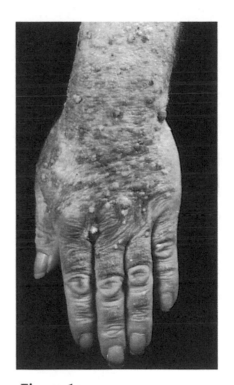

Figure 1a

The sign of Leser–Trélat.
This is the 'explosive' onset of multiple, small seborrhoeic keratoses. In this patient with adenocarcinoma of the stomach there were myriads of seborrhoeic keratoses on the arms and hands.

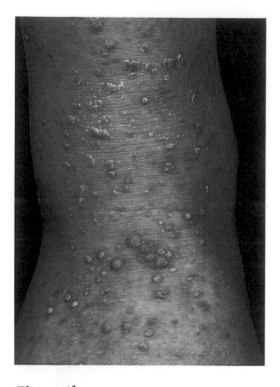

Figure 1b

The sign of Leser–Trélat.
Seborrhoeic keratoses also developed on
the legs.

Investigations

Hb: 8.9 g/dl (11.5–15.5 g/dl), WCC: 11.9×10^9/l
($4.0–11.0 \times 10^9$/l), plts: 576×10^9/l ($150–450 \times 10^9$/l), ESR: 74 mm/hr (1–10 mm/hr).

Upper GI endoscopy: There was a 1 cm gastric
ulcer in the antral region of the stomach.

Gastric biopsy histopathology demonstrated
poorly differentiated gastric adenocarcinoma
of the diffuse type with numerous 'signet-
ring' forms (Figure 1e).

CT abdomen and chest: There was thickening of the posteroinferior aspect of the gastric
antral wall and widespread regional
lymphadenopathy.

Skin histopathology: Biopsy of axillary skin
demonstrated confluent hyperkeratosis,
papillomatosis and mild acanthosis, consistent with acanthosis nigricans. Biopsy of a
keratotic papule from the leg showed a
sharply defined exophytic lesion composed of
broad columns of basaloid cells with papillomatosis and hyperkeratosis, consistent with
a seborrhoeic keratosis.

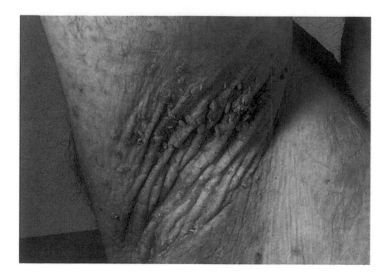

Figure 1c

Malignant acanthosis nigricans.
There are marked changes in the
right axilla with hyperpigmented
velvety thickening and warty
excrescences.

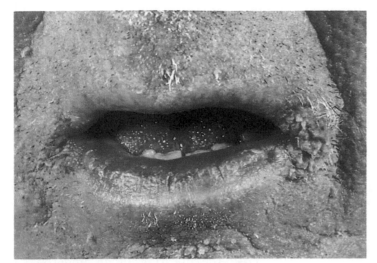

Figure 1d

Malignant acanthosis nigricans.
There is marked papillomatosis at the commissures of the mouth.

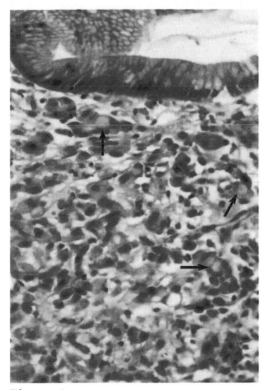

Figure 1e

Adenocarcinoma of the stomach.
Histopathology of stomach biopsy (H&E, high power). The gastric mucosa is infiltrated by poorly differentiated adenocarcinoma with 'signet-ring' cell formation (*arrows*).

Diagnosis

Adenocarcinoma of the stomach with the sign of Leser–Trélat and malignant acanthosis nigricans.

Treatment and progress

The patient underwent six cycles of combination chemotherapy using epirubicin, cisplatin and 5-fluorouracil. After three cycles, the acanthosis nigricans had resolved and the seborrhoeic keratoses had reduced in number. A repeat CT after chemotherapy showed reduction of the mediastinal and abdominal lymphadenopathy. Despite an initial encouraging response to treatment the patient died 10 months after presentation.

Comment

The sign of Leser–Trélat is the association of eruptive, pruritic seborrhoeic keratoses with occult internal malignancy, most usually adenocarcinoma of the colon, breast or stomach. As in our case, the condition is often accompanied by acanthosis nigricans (AN), which, when occurring as a paraneoplastic phenomenon, is also most commonly associated with an underlying adenocarcinoma. These dermatoses may precede, follow or develop concurrently with the presentation of the cancer and usually reflect metastatic disease and poor prognosis. Some reports of Leser–Trélat/malignant AN have presented in conjunction with other paraneoplastic dermatoses, such as hypertrichosis lanugosa and acquired ichthyosis.

The cutaneous changes of malignant AN are more florid than those of AN associated with insulin resistance. In malignant AN, as in our case, gross eruptive papillomatosis of the major flexures and mouth (both commissures and oral cavity) tends to occur often in association with a palmo–plantar keratoderma.

Histologically, both seborrhoeic keratoses and AN are characterised by non-inflammatory, epidermal hyperproliferation. Evidence suggests that there is a humoral link between internal malignancy and the appearance of seborrhoeic keratoses and AN. The epidermal growth factor receptor (EGFR) mediates epidermal proliferation; EGFR-stimulated keratinocytes produce transforming growth factor-α (TGF-α), which can, in an autocrine fashion, further stimulate keratinocyte division. It has been suggested that internal malignancy may elaborate TGF-α, which can induce epidermal changes. Cytokine-driven epidermal growth may be modulated by the local milieu, thus papillomatosis develops in flexural skin while seborrhoeic keratoses develop on non-flexural skin.

Learning points

1. The presentation of multiple, eruptive, pruritic seborrhoeic keratoses (sign of Leser–Trélat) should raise the question of an underlying malignancy.
2. Malignant acanthosis nigricans (AN) often occurs concurrently.
3. Other cutaneous signs of internal malignancy include: acquired ichthyosis, hypertrichosis lanugosa, dermatomyositis, erythema gyratum repens and paraneoplastic pemphigus.

Reference

Poole S, Fenske NA. Cutaneous markers of internal malignancy. *J Am Acad Dermatol* 1993; 28: 147–64.

See also case number 42.

Case 2
Annular lesions on the face of a neonate

History

A 1-month-old baby girl was referred with a 5-day history of a facial rash. The child was otherwise well, breast-feeding successfully and gaining weight appropriately. The pregnancy had been uncomplicated. The child's parents were both well with no significant past medical history.

Clinical features

The baby appeared well. There were several raised, annular hyperpigmented lesions on the face (Figures 2a, b). Similar lesions were also observed in the scalp. Discrete erythematous macules were present on the palms and soles. Atrophic hyperpigmented lesions were seen on the back. The heart rate was 120 beats per minute and regular.

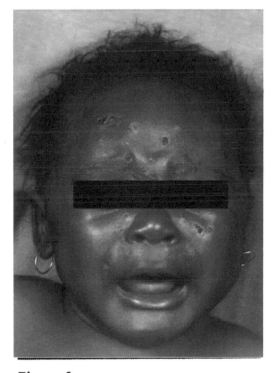

Figure 2a

Neonatal lupus erythematosus.
There are multiple annular, hyperpigmented lesions scattered over the face and scalp.

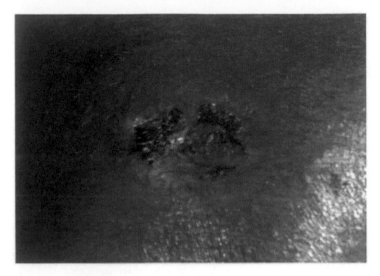

Figure 2b

Neonatal lupus erythematosus.
Close-up of an annular lesion on the
forehead demonstrates central hyperpigmentation and atrophy.

Investigations

Hb: 10.2 g/dl (11.5–15.5 g/dl), WCC: 6.9 ×
10^9/l (4.0–11.0 × 10^9/l), plts: 106 × 10^9/l
(150–450 × 10^9/l).

ECG: normal sinus rhythm.

ANA: negative.

ENA: Ro positive; La negative.

Skin histopathology: Biopsy of an annular
lesion demonstrated mild hyperkeratosis, an
interface dermatitis with basal vacuolation
and lymphocyte exocytosis (Figure 2c).

Skin direct immunofluorescence: negative.

Mother's ANA: 1 in 10.

Mother's ENA: Ro positive.

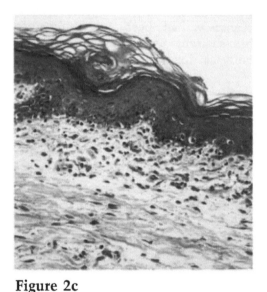

Figure 2c

Neonatal lupus erythematosus.
Skin histopathology (H&E, medium power).
There is an interface dermatitis with basal
vacuolation and lymphocytic exocytosis.
There is overlying hyperkeratosis.

Diagnosis

Neonatal lupus erythematosus.

Treatment and progress

The child's cutaneous lesions cleared over the next 3 weeks using a mild topical corticosteroid. There was some post-inflammatory hyperpigmentation and minimal residual atrophic scarring. Six months after presentation a repeated ENA was negative, showing loss of the circulating Ro antibody.

The mother was advised that her subsequent pregnancies should be closely monitored. Despite this recommendation, 6 years later she represented with a second baby girl born 2 months earlier following an unsupervised pregnancy. The new baby had, like her older sister, a number of inflammatory lesions on the skin of her face. Investigations revealed a positive Ro antibody. She was otherwise well, with no cardiac problems. The cutaneous lesions settled over the next few weeks with the use of a mild topical corticosteroid.

Comment

Neonatal lupus erythematosus (NLE) is a lupus syndrome caused by autoantibodies that are passively acquired by the fetus from the maternal circulation. The majority of infants with NLE exhibit cutaneous and/or cardiac disease, although other manifestations have been described. Females seem to be affected more frequently than males, particularly by NLE skin disease. These skin lesions may be present at birth but usually develop days to weeks and sometimes months after delivery. Cutaneous NLE may be precipitated or exacerbated by UV light exposure and there are reported cases of cutaneous NLE being precipitated by phototherapy for hyperbilirubinaemia.

NLE skin lesions are both clinically and histopathologically similar to those of subacute cutaneous LE, which is also characterized by a positive ENA, usually anti-Ro. Lesions, which are commonly found on the face, begin as erythematous macules, which enlarge into annular patches and plaques often with fine overlying scale. Spontaneous resolution within weeks is usual, with transient dyspigmentation, telangiectasis and epidermal atrophy. Histologically the lesions of NLE are characterized by vacuolar degeneration of the basal keratinocytes and a lymphocytic infiltrate in the upper dermis.

Although our patient had no demonstrable cardiac problems, complete heart block (CHB) occurs in approximately 50% of cases of NLE. A slow fetal heart rate noticed late in pregnancy provides the first clue of CHB. Fetal echocardiography confirms heart block by demonstrating slow ventricular contraction occurring independently of the atria. Mortality rates in infants with CHB may be as high as 20%. Other manifestations of NLE include anaemia and transient thrombocytopenia, as in our patient. Hepatomegaly may occur, which is secondary either to extramedullary haematopoiesis or to congestive heart failure.

Learning points

1. The association of annular skin lesions and complete heart block in an infant is strongly suggestive of neonatal lupus erythematosus (NLE).
2. NLE is caused by Ro autoantibodies (occasionally La) transferred from the maternal circulation to the fetus.
3. The mother should be investigated for lupus erythematosus and be warned that NLE may develop in future pregnancies.

Ro autoantibodies are present in approximately 80% of NLE patients and in 90% of their mothers. La autoantibodies are observed less frequently. Maternally derived autoantibodies appear to play a direct role in the pathogenesis of the NLE skin disease, an association supported by the simultaneous clearance of the dermatosis and maternally acquired antibodies at about 6 months of age.

Reference

McCauliffe DP. Neonatal lupus erythematosus: a transplacentally acquired autoimmune disorder. *Semin Dermatol* 1995; 14: 47–53.

See also case number 18.

Case 3
A warty plaque on the sole of the foot

History

A 62-year-old Indian man presented with a warty plaque on the sole of the right foot. The lesion had first developed as a small papule 40 years previously and had gradually increased in size over the intervening years. During his twenties he had worked as an agricultural labourer in India, frequently walking barefoot. One year prior to presentation the lesion had become very painful and had enlarged further.

Clinical findings

Examination revealed a 6 cm × 5 cm verrucous plaque on the plantar aspect of his right foot. It was indurated with a warty, keratotic surface and an irregular outline (Figure 3a). No regional lymph nodes were palpable. General examination was unremarkable.

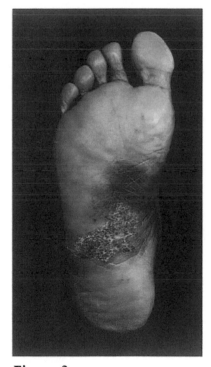

Figure 3a

Tuberculosis verrucosa cutis.
A large, warty, hyperpigmented plaque is present on the sole of the right foot.

Investigations

FBC, U&E, LFT, immunoglobulins: all normal.

Skin histopathology: Biopsy of the plaque demonstrated marked pseudoepitheliomatous hyperplasia of the epidermis with hyperkeratosis and an underlying dense inflammatory cell infiltrate including the presence of necrotizing granulomata with giant cells. Special stains for mycobacteria and fungi were negative (Figure 3b).

Chest x-ray: normal.

Heaf test: grade IV reaction.

Tissue culture: *Mycobacterium tuberculosis* was cultured from lesional skin after 4 weeks.

Diagnosis

Tuberculosis verrucosa cutis.

Treatment and progress

Multidrug therapy was administered for 2 months (rifampicin 600 mg/day, isoniazid 400 mg/day and pyrazinamide 2 g/day) followed by rifampicin and isoniazid alone for the next 2 months. At 6-month follow-up there was complete resolution of the lesion.

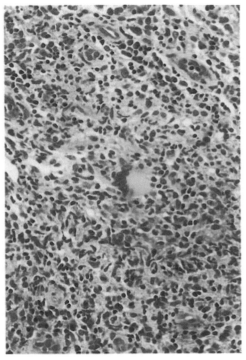

Figure 3b

Tuberculosis verrucosa cutis.
Skin histopathology (H&E, high power). The dermal inflammation includes an epithelioid cell granuloma with a central multinucleated Langerhans giant cell. Caseation necrosis is not present in this granuloma.

Comment

Tuberculosis verrucosa cutis is caused by exogenous inoculation of tubercle bacilli into the skin of individuals with a pre-existing moderately high degree of immunity to the organism. In tropical climates, tuberculosis verrucosa cutis is generally a disease affecting children or young adults who contract the bacteria by walking barefoot or sitting on ground contaminated with tuberculous sputum. In such cases, lesions develop on the soles of the feet, as in our case, or on the buttocks. It may also occur as an occupational hazard on the hands of medical personnel working in the autopsy room. The lesion is typically asymptomatic and starts as a small papule or papulopustule with a purple inflammatory halo. Deep clefts and fissures extend into the brownish-red underlying base. Progression to a warty or hyperkeratotic plaque usually follows. The lesion is firm and may occasionally discharge pus. Regional lymph nodes are not commonly enlarged.

Clinically, the differential diagnosis includes other unusual infections such as chromoblastomycosis, primary sporotrichosis and lesions caused by atypical mycobacteria. Inflammatory dermatoses including psoriasis, lichen simplex chronicus and hypertrophic lichen planus may also mimic this condition.

Histopathological assessment rarely reveals the presence of acid-fast bacilli since the lesion commonly contains only small numbers of organisms. However, culture of skin usually yields *M. tuberculosis*. Standard anti-tuberculous therapy is the treatment of choice and most lesions resolve after 4–5 months.

Learning points

1. Tuberculosis verrucosa cutis is caused by inoculation of tubercle bacilli into the skin of individuals with good TB immunity.
2. Clinically it is characterized by a warty plaque found most commonly on the sole, buttock or hand.
3. A skin biopsy for histology and culture is necessary to establish the diagnosis.

Reference

Sehgall VN, Srivastava G, Khurana VK et al. An appraisal of epidemiologic, clinical bacteriologic, histopathologic and immunologic parameters in cutaneous tuberculosis. *Int J Dermatol* 1987; 26: 521–6.

See also case number 24.

Case 4
Dystrophic nails and lethargy

History

A 54-year-old woman presented with a 1-year history of painless dystrophy of all 10 finger nails. She described her nails as becoming brittle and fragile whilst some were lost altogether. Over this period she also complained of increasing lethargy.

Clinical findings

There was nail plate thinning and longitudinal ridging of most of the finger nails. Three of them were absent, the nail beds being pale and firm (Figure 4a). The nail folds were normal. Examination of the rest of the skin was unremarkable. General examination revealed peripheral oedema.

Investigations

Hb: 9.7 g/dl (11.5–15.5 g/dl), WCC: 6.6×10^9/l ($4.0–11.0 \times 10^9$/l), plts: 286×10^9/l ($150–450 \times 10^9$/l). ESR: 64 mm/hr (1–10 mm/hr). Blood film: rouleaux formations.

Serum creatinine: 139 µmol/l (40–120 µmol/l), albumin: 26 g/l (35–50 g/l), calcium: 2.64 mmol/l (2.20–2.60 mmol/l).

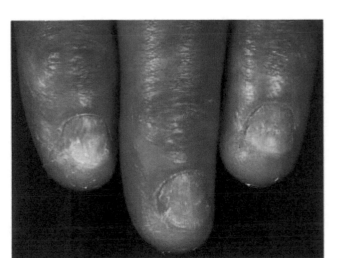

Figure 4a

Systemic amyloidosis.
There is loss of the nail plate (anonychia) in three fingers.

Skin histopathology: Biopsy of a nail bed revealed eosinophilic amorphous deposits which stained with Congo red and displayed apple-green birefringence under polarized light (Figure 4b).

IgG, IgA, IgM: all reduced.

Serum protein electrophoresis: IgG-λ monoclonal paraprotein, 9.6 g/l.

Urinary Bence-Jones protein analysis: positive.

Skeletal radiographic survey: multiple lytic lesions (Figure 4c).

Bone marrow biopsy: >20% plasma cells, many showing abnormal forms.

Renal histopathology: extensive glomerular deposition of amyloid (Figure 4d).

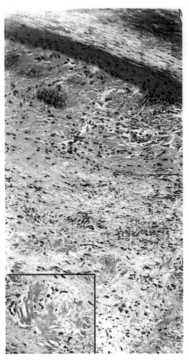

Figure 4b

Systemic amyloidosis.
Nail bed histopathology (H&E, low power). There is upper dermal deposition of eosinophilic material. *Insert* (Congo red, high power): positive staining of dermal deposit with Congo red confirms amyloid.

Diagnosis

Myeloma-associated systemic amyloidosis.

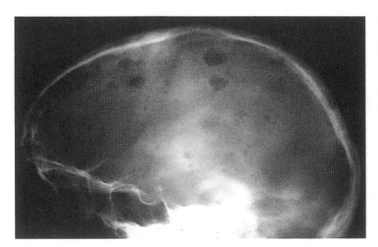

Figure 4c

Multiple myeloma.
The patient's skull x-ray revealed numerous lytic lesions. Systemic amyloidosis developed secondary to multiple myeloma.

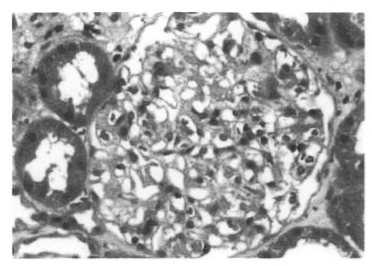

Figure 4d

Systemic amyloidosis.
Renal histopathology (H&E, high power). There is an enlarged glomerulus showing mesangial expansion by eosinophilic hyaline material that was confirmed as amyloid on Congo red staining.

Treatment and progress

An elevated 24-hour urinary protein analysis demonstrated nephrotic syndrome [5.6 g/24 hours (normal: <0.15 g/24 hrs)], and a renal biopsy revealed the presence of extensive glomerular amyloid deposits (Figure 4d). The patient received 6 cycles of C-VAMP chemotherapy (cyclophosphamide, vincristine, doxorubicin and methylprednisolone) but with little reduction in paraproteinaemia. She developed worsening renal function and congestive cardiac failure (secondary to presumed cardiac amyloid) and died 1 year after diagnosis.

Comment

The amyloidoses are a heterogenous group of disorders characterized by the extracellular deposition of amyloid, a fibrillar protein arranged in a beta-pleated sheet. With light microscopy, amyloid appears as an eosinophilic amorphous substance but demonstrates apple-green birefringence on Congo red staining when viewed with polarized light.

The clinical manifestations of the amyloidoses depend both on the underlying disease pathogenesis and on the type of amyloid fibril deposited. In myeloma-associated systemic amyloidosis immunoglobulin light chains act as precursors to the amyloid fibril protein, termed 'amyloid L' (AL). Most of these immunoglobulins are of the lambda (λ) type, derived from serum immunoglobulins originating from a clonal plasma cell dyscrasia.

The association of multiple myeloma with systemic amyloidosis can result in striking cutaneous signs from amyloid deposition in the skin. Petechiae, ecchymoses and macroglossia are manifestations most readily associated with systemic amyloid; however, papules, plaques, bullae and, as in our case, nail dystrophy are also recognized. The nail abnormalities seen in patients with systemic amyloidosis are heterogenous depending on the location and size of the amyloid deposits within the nail apparatus. Brittleness, increased fragility, longitudinal ridging, onycholysis and subungual striations have been described. Partial or, as in our case, complete anonychia can also occur. Our case illustrates the importance of histopathology

The presence of systemic amyloidosis in multiple myeloma can result in considerable morbidity and is a major cause of death in plasma cell malignancies. As in our case, renal involvement can cause nephrotic syndrome and renal failure, while cardiac involvement will lead to heart failure. Treatment of amyloidosis is directed at managing the underlying myeloma, and patients who respond to chemotherapy may proceed to haematopoietic stem cell transplantation.

in the diagnosis of nail disorders. In the absence of other relevant physical signs, the diagnosis of systemic amyloidosis was reached through biopsy of the nail bed.

Reference

Daoud MS, Lust JA, Kyle RA et al. Monoclonal gammopathies and associated skin disorders. *J Am Acad Dermatol* 1999; 40: 507–35.

See also case number 7, 38.

Case 5
Stretchy skin

History

A 14-year-old boy presented to the dermatology department with hand eczema and mild acne. Incidentally, he mentioned that he had easily extensible skin. He also admitted to having hypermobile joints and complained of bilateral knee and ankle pain. His past medical history included a spontaneous left-sided pneumothorax and dislocation of the right shoulder following minimal trauma. There was no family history of hyperextensible skin or hypermobile joints.

Clinical findings

The patient was tall, slim and marfanoid. His height was 176 cm and his arm span was 182.5 cm. He was markedly loose-jointed with a 9/9 Beighton score (used to assess extent of hypermobility) (Figure 5a). He had a single papyraceous scar on the left knee. Blood pressure was 148/80 and on auscultation there was a systolic click at the apex. There was evidence of hyperelastic skin at the elbows, knees and neck (Figure 5b). There was no joint tenderness or synovitis. His thoracic spine demonstrated increased spine kyphosis. Ophthalmological examination was normal.

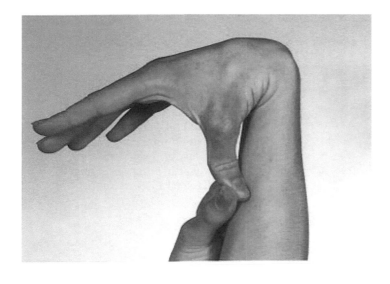

Figure 5a

Ehlers–Danlos syndrome.
There is hypermobility of the thumb joints. Joint laxity can lead to premature osteoarthritis.

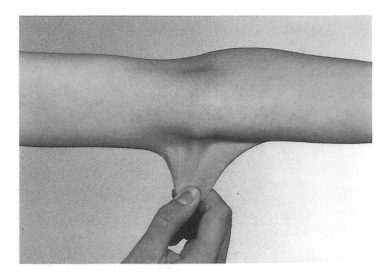

Figure 5b
Ehlers–Danlos syndrome.
The skin over the elbow is hyperextensible. The elastic recoil of the skin is normal.

Investigations

Electrocardiograph: normal.

Echocardiogram: mitral valve prolapse.

Electron microscopy of skin: Loosely packed bundles of collagen were seen throughout the superficial dermis. In the mid and deep dermis collagen fibrils of variable diameter were observed as well as cauliflower-like collagen fibrils (Figure 5c). Some of the elastin fibres were also noted to be fragmented.

Diagnosis

Classical Ehlers–Danlos syndrome (type I/II).

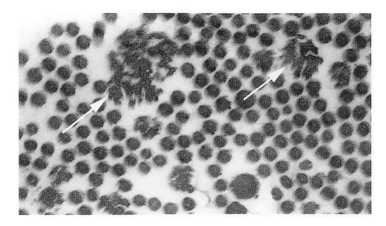

Figure 5c
Ehlers–Danlos syndrome.
Electron micrograph of the mid-dermis. The collagen fibres are of various diameter and there are numerous 'cauliflower' forms (arrowed), features that are typically seen in classical EDS.

Treatment and progress

The patient was advised that this mild form of Ehlers–Danlos syndrome should not greatly affect his health apart from a risk of further shoulder dislocation, spontaneous pneumothorax and late-onset osteoarthritis. He has a 50% chance of onward transmission of the syndrome to his children.

Comment

Ehlers–Danlos syndrome (EDS) is a collection of inherited connective tissue disorders unified by a susceptibility to hyperextensible skin and joint laxity. The sub-types were originally described according to their clinical features, however, the current classification is based on an understanding of the molecular pathogenesis of each sub-group. In the majority of EDS sub-groups the molecular defect involves the synthesis, structure or function of one of the fibrillar collagens (collagen types I, III and V). Variation in molecular defects leads to great clinical heterogeneity between different EDS sub-groups: for many patients the symptoms are so minimal that they remain undiagnosed, whereas vascular EDS (type IV) may lead to premature death due to fatal arterial rupture.

The cardinal manifestations of EDS include hyperextensible, soft skin, atrophic scars, easy bruising, joint hypermobility and variable involvement of internal organs. The skin is hyperextensible but retains its normal elastic recoil. Scars develop over trauma-prone sites, such as elbows and knees, and become apparent once the child begins to crawl or walk. The atrophic nature of these scars leads to a papyraceous or 'cigarette paper' appearance. Fibroid lumps (molluscoid pseudotumours) measuring 2–3 cm may arise at sites of repetitive trauma. Subcutaneous nodules, which show calcification on x-ray,

***

Learning points

1. Ehlers–Danlos syndrome (EDS) represents a collection of inherited disorders of connective tissue resulting from mutations of collagen genes or enzymes that catalyse collagen post-translational modification.
2. Clinically, EDS is characterized by joint laxity and cutaneous signs, particularly hyperextensible skin with a doughy texture, papyraceous scars and molluscoid pseudotumours.
3. Patients with classical EDS (I and II) are prone to mitral valve prolapse, spontaneous pneumothorax and joint dislocations.

***

develop in a third of cases along the shins or forearms. These lesions probably represent subcutaneous fat lobules that have undergone fibrosis and calcification due to the loss of blood supply. Thin skin and bruising are more prominent in vascular EDS and some individuals have acrogeric appearances of face, hands and feet. Other dermatological features include epicanthic folds (more common in EDS type I), keratosis pilaris-like changes around the elbows and knees, and pedal peizogenic papules. Elastosis perforans serpiginosa is seen typically in vascular EDS.

EDS types I and II are the commonest variants and are known collectively as 'classical' EDS. Electron microscopy of dermal collagen fibrils in affected individuals often shows gross abnormalities of fibril shape and size, suggesting a defect in fibril-logenesis. Abnormalities have been described in type V collagen and investigators have demonstrated significant linkage to *COL5A1*. Clinically, classical EDS has fairly mild manifestations, as in our case. As well as the cutaneous features described above, a significant number of individuals have cardiac defects, most commonly mitral valve prolapse. However, most morbidity in classical EDS arises from the susceptiblity to joint hypermobility leading to dislocations and a premature onset of osteoarthritis.

There is no specific therapy for classical EDS, however appropriate advice can limit orthopaedic complications and arthritis.

Reference

Burrows NP. The molecular genetics of the Ehlers–Danlos syndrome. *Clin Exp Dermatol* 1999; 24: 99–106.

See also case number 49.

Case 6
Chronic scaling of the scalp

History

A 21-year-old medical student presented with a 5-year history of a pruritic scaling eruption of the scalp. This was initially diagnosed as a staphylococcal folliculitis, since *Staphylococcus aureus* had been cultured on several occasions. However, there had been little improvement with topical and systemic antimicrobial therapy and so further investigations were suggested.

Clinical findings

Examination revealed a diffuse scalp dermatosis characterized by scaling, crusting, erythema and induration. There was no scarring or hair loss. After the removal of overlying scale it was possible to see individual, brown, purpuric, crusted papules (Figure 6a). A few similar papules were seen along the alae nasi and in the conchi of the ears. General medical examination was normal.

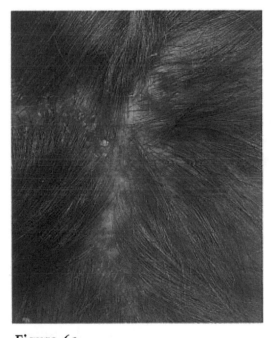

Figure 6a

Langerhans cell hystiocytosis.
There is crusting and erythema of the scalp without alopecia. Removal of the scale revealed petechial haemorrhages.

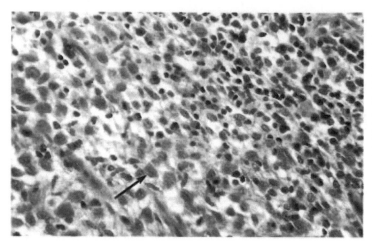

Figure 6b

Langerhans cell hystiocytosis.
Skin histopathology (H&E, high power). Within the dermis there is a mixed infiltrate consisting of numerous Langerhans cell histiocytes, eosinophils and smaller numbers of lymphocytes. The Langerhans cells are large ovoid histiocytes with abundant eosinophilic cytoplasm and indented 'coffee bean' nuclei (arrow).

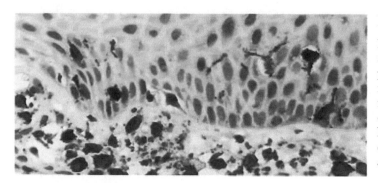

Figure 6c

Langerhans cell hystiocytosis.
Skin immunohistopathology (high power): S100 immunostaining of interfollicular skin reveals large immunoreactive cells in the upper dermis, which are Langerhans cell histiocytes. S100-positive dendritic cells in the epidermis are melanocytes and Langerhans cells.

Investigations

Skin histopathology: Biopsy of the scalp demonstrated dense nodular aggregates of histiocytic cells in the mid and upper dermis (Figure 6b). Immunohistochemistry revealed that the histiocytic cells stained positively for CD1a and S100 (Figure 6c).

FBC: normal, U&E: normal, LFT: normal, immunoglobulins: normal.

Chest x-ray: normal.

Skull x-ray: normal.

Abdominal ultrasound: no organomegaly.

Bone marrow biopsy: normal.

Diagnosis

Langerhans cell histiocytosis.

Treatment and progress

Topical nitrogen mustard was used daily to the scalp for one month, resulting in complete resolution of the eruption. Further staging investigations showed no evidence of systemic involvement by Langerhans cell histiocytosis. The patient was followed up for a number of years without relapse. Twenty years following presentation he remains free of disease.

Comment

The histiocytoses are a group of disorders characterized by a benign or malignant proliferation of histiocytic cells. Langerhans cell histiocytosis (LCH), assigned to class I of the histiocytosis classification system, appears to be a reactive condition in which cells with the phenotype of Langerhans cells accumulate in various organs, including skin, bone, lymph nodes, lungs and pituitary. Class II includes histiocytoses of mononuclear phagocytes other than Langerhans cells, while class III comprises malignant histiocytic disorders.

Skin is frequently the site of first presentation of LCH and often simulates seborrhoeic dermatitis with irritation, erythema and scaling in the scalp, groins, submammary flexures and nasolabial folds. An erosive intertrigo in the groins, axillae and perianal region is also a recognized pattern of presentation in both children and adults. Close examination of the eruption of LCH often reveals the presence of petechial haemorrhages in involved skin, an important sign in the recognition of the condition.

Histologically LCH is characterized by sheets of large ovoid histiocytic cells containing an indented or 'coffee bean' nucleus. The cells are usually present in the upper dermis and sometimes invade the epidermis. There is usually an admixture of other inflammatory cells including eosinophils. The Langerhans cells stain positively for CD1a and S100 while electron microscopy reveals the presence of Birbeck granules.

Overall morbidity and mortality in LCH is related to the number of tissues involved and the presence of organ dysfunction. Prognosis is best in single-organ disease, such as in our case. Internal involvement is identified with conventional imaging techniques and also with radioimmunoimaging utilizing radio-labelled monoclonal antibodies to CD1a, a marker for Langerhans cells.

Treatment of LCH depends on the extent and severity of the disease. In skin involvement alone, topical treatment with nitrogen mustard is effective. Psoralen-UVA (PUVA) photochemotherapy may be useful for those patients who do not tolerate topical nitrogen mustard or who fail to respond adequately. In multi-system LCH, where there is evidence of organ dysfunction, systemic chemotherapy is indicated using prednisolone alone or in combination with vinca alkaloids.

Learning points

1. LCH of the skin can mimic seborrhoeic dermatitis with involvement of the scalp, flexures and nasolabial folds. A biopsy is necessary to establish the diagnosis.
2. Histologically cutaneous LCH is characterized by an upper dermal infiltrate of histiocytic cells. These Langerhans histiocytes demonstrate positive immunoreactivity for S100 and CD1a.
3. The diagnosis of cutaneous LCH requires further investigation to exclude systemic involvement.

Reference

1. Chu A. Langerhans cell histiocytosis. *Aust J Dermatol* 2001; 42: 237–42.

See also case number 19.

Case 7
Generalized papular thickening of the skin

History

A 65-year-old man presented with a 6-month history of gradual thickening and stiffening of his skin. In many places this was associated with a widespread, confluent, papular eruption. He was unable to open his mouth fully and the movements of his elbows and knees were restricted. He was referred to our department when his skin disorder resulted in difficulty getting out of a chair and walking up and down stairs.

Clinical features

Examination of his facial skin revealed hyperpigmented, sclerodermatous changes with numerous monomorphic papules, particularly on the cheeks and forehead and behind the ears (Figures 7a, b). In places, the papules were arranged in a linear configuration. There was microstomia (Figure 7c). A similar scleroderma with lichenoid papules also involved the trunk and limbs (Figure 7d). There were flexion deformities of the elbows and knees resulting in functional disability (Figure 7e).

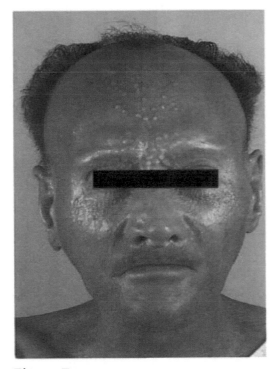

Figure 7a

Scleromyxoedema.
Scleroderma of the face with multiple skin-coloured papules on the forehead, cheeks and eyelids.

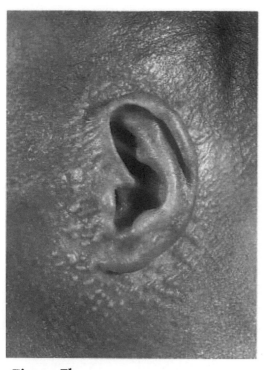

Figure 7b

Scleromyxoedema.
Waxy, lichenoid papules around the left
ear, some arranged in a characteristic
linear pattern.

Investigations

Hb: 12.7 g/dl (11.5–15.5 g/dl), WCC: 9.8 ×
10^9/l (4.0–11.0 × 10^9/l), eos: 3.1 × 10^9/l
(0.1–0.4 × 10^9/l), plts: 259 × 10^9/l (150–450 ×
10^9/l). ESR: 69 mm/hr (1–10 mm/hr).

Serum protein electrophoresis: IgG-λ
paraprotein of 22 g/l.

Urine Bence-Jones protein: positive at a
concentration of 7.7 mg/l.

Skin histopathology: There was thickened
reticular dermis showing a prominent proliferation of fibroblasts. There was a moderate
perivascular inflammatory cell infiltrate.
Alcian blue staining demonstrated excessive
mucin deposition.

Bone marrow biopsy: 7% clonal plasma cell
population (IgG-λ positive).

Skeletal x-ray survey: normal.

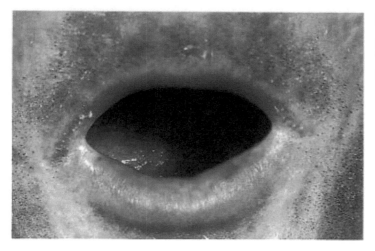

Figure 7c

Scleromyxoedema.
The disorder may result in
microstomia.

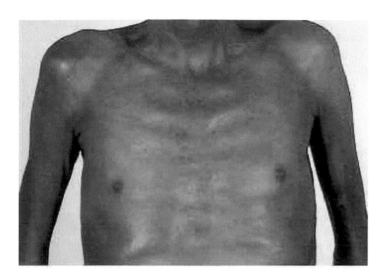

Figure 7d

Scleromyxoedema.
There are generalized
sclerodermatous changes with
hyperpigmentation.

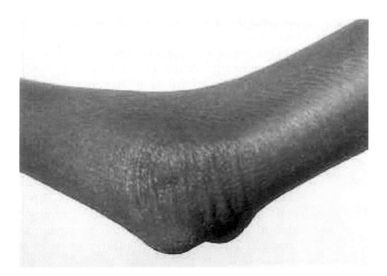

Figure 7e

Scleromyxoedema.
Fixed flexion deformities constitute a
serious functional disability.

Diagnosis

Scleromyxoedema.

Treatment and progress

Prednisolone was given at a dose of 40 mg/day, but there was no cutaneous or haematological improvement. Subsequently, the patient underwent a 3-month trial of psoralen-UVA (PUVA) photochemotherapy but the skin changes remained unaltered. He thereafter developed a severe proximal myopathy confirmed by myopathic changes on electromyography. Total skin electron-beam radiotherapy was administered, again without benefit. Latterly, melphalan was given, with some reduction in the parapro-teinaemia but no apparent beneficial effect on the dermatosis. Ten years after presentation the patient died from unrelated causes.

Comment

The term 'scleromyxoedema' is used for a sclerotic variant of papular mucinosis that develops into a chronic, disabling condition. Scleromyxoedema is associated with many systemic disorders, most consistently with paraproteinaemia in which the monoclonal gammopathy is usually IgG with λ light chains. Although a plasmacytosis may be found in the bone marrow, the monoclonal gammopathy progresses to multiple myeloma in only 10% of cases. Other systemic manifestations that have also been reported include myopathy, eosinophilia, arthritis and central nervous system disorders, including coma.

Scleromyxoedema is characterized by a widespread, symmetrical eruption of small, firm, waxy, closely spaced papules that are located on the face, hands, forearms, neck, upper trunk and thighs. Papules are commonly arranged in a linear pattern while the remaining skin is shiny and resembles scleroderma. The mucous membranes and the scalp are not involved. As the condition progresses, erythematous and infiltrated plaques may occur with skin stiffening, sclerodactyly and decreased mobility of the mouth and joints. Telangiectases and calcinosis are always absent.

Histologically, the skin shows a diffuse deposit of mucin in the upper and mid reticular dermis, an increased collagen deposition and a marked proliferation of irregularly arranged fibroblasts. Although the exact pathogenesis of scleromyxoedema is not known, various hypotheses exist. It has been proposed that the paraprotein acts as an autoantibody and directly stimulates fibroblast proliferation and mucin deposition in the skin.

Treatment of scleromyxoedema is often disappointing. Melphalan may improve the condition but there is evidence that such patients are at increased risk of a secondary haematological malignancy. PUVA and total skin electron-beam radiotherapy have been reported to reduce skin thickening but do not influence extracutaneous manifestations of the disease. However, there have been recent encouraging reports of the use of extracorporeal photopheresis, intravenous immunoglobulin, thalidomide and autologous haematopoietic stem cell transplantation.

Learning points

1. A diagnosis of scleromyxoedema should be considered in a patient presenting with generalized scleroderma and widespread waxy, lichenoid papules.
2. Scleromyxoedema is commonly associated with an IgG monoclonal gammopathy producing λ light chains.
3. Joint contractures and an associated myopathy often result in significant functional disability.

Reference

Rongioletti F, Rebora A. Updated classification of papular mucinosis, lichen myxedematosus, and scleromyxedema. *J Am Acad Dermatol* 2001: 44; 273–81.

See also case numbers 4, 21, 26.

Case 8
Flexural erythema following chemotherapy

History

A 39-year-old man with myelodysplastic syndrome was admitted for an allogeneic haematopoietic stem cell transplant. He received conditioning chemotherapy with busulfan and cyclophosphamide, and, following stem cell infusion, was given methotrexate and cyclophosphamide as graft-versus-host-disease prophylaxis. Two days following the transplant (nine days after first exposure to chemotherapy) the patient developed an eruption involving the flexural and acral skin.

Clinical features

Clinical examination revealed a striking symmetrical eruption consisting of well-defined, deep-red oedematous plaques in the axillae, antecubital fossae and groins (Figures 8a, b). The scrotum also demonstrated

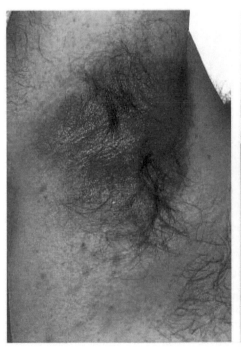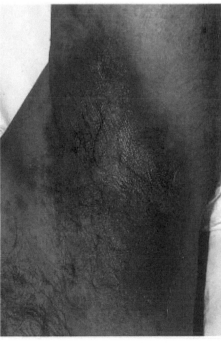

Figure 8a

Eccrine squamous syringometaplasia. There is a symmetrical, well-defined erythema in the axillae.

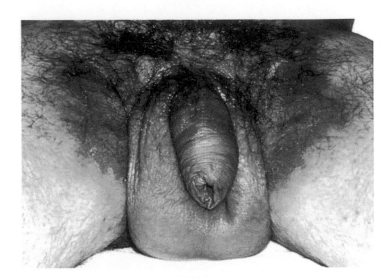

Figure 8b

Eccrine squamous syringometaplasia.
There is confluent erythema and
oedema of the groins, scrotum and
penis. The eruption is typically well-
demarcated.

confluent erythema. The palms and soles
displayed a more subtle erythema. The
patient was afebrile. There was no regional
lymphadenopathy.

Investigations

Mycology: negative.

Bacteriology: negative.

Skin histopathology: Biopsy of the axillary
skin showed a normal epidermis except for
occasional necrotic keratinocytes. There was
mild oedema of the upper dermis. The
epithelium of the superficial sweat ducts was
expanded with multiple layers of enlarged
epithelioid cells consistent with squamous
metaplasia. There was no associated inflammatory infiltrate (Figure 8c).

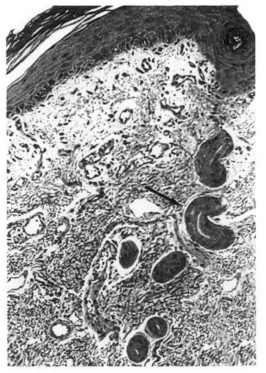

Figure 8c

Eccrine squamous syringometaplasia.
Skin histopathology (H&E, medium power).
There is marked squamous metaplasia of the
acrosyringium and secretory coils of the eccrine
gland (arrow).

Diagnosis

Eccrine squamous syringometaplasia.

Treatment and progress

The patient was treated with a potent topical steroid. The eruption resolved within 5 days. There was no relapse.

Comment

Eccrine squamous syringometaplasia (ESS) is a tissue reaction pattern observed occasionally as an incidental finding in a number of cutaneous pathologies (eg ulcer margins). However, a distinct eruption of ESS has been described in patients with haematological malignancy who have received pre-transplantation chemotherapy and a stem cell transplantation. As in our patient, other reported cases have demonstrated a flexural erythema, particularly marked in the axillae and groins, which was characterized histologically by squamous metaplasia of the eccrine sweat glands. In contrast to other acute dermatoses following chemotherapy and haematopoietic stem cell transplantation (eg graft-versus-host disease), the eruption of ESS is usually self-limiting and without systemic upset.

ESS and neutrophilic eccrine hidradenitis are both cutaneous reactions to the toxic effects of chemotherapeutic agents on the eccrine gland. ESS is at the non-inflammatory end of the spectrum and neutrophilic eccrine hidradenitis is at the inflammatory end. However, overlap cases have been reported sharing pathological and cutaneous features. In ESS it has been proposed that the toxic effect of the chemotherapeutic agent induces squamous metaplasia of the eccrine

acrosyringium and duct and an irritant reaction on the skin surface. The distribution of the eruption is explained by an exaggeration of drug toxicity in flexural areas secondary to friction, local temperature and density of eccrine glands.

Typically, the dermatosis of ESS is asymptomatic and resolves spontaneously in 7–10 days.

Learning points

1. The occurrence of a flexural eruption in a patient undergoing chemotherapy for haematological malignancy should suggest a diagnosis of eccrine squamous syringometaplasia (ESS), once an infective intertrigo has been excluded.
2. The histological changes are diagnostic and so a skin biopsy is mandatory.
3. Chemotherapy-induced ESS is usually self-limiting.

Reference

Valks R, Fraga J, Porras-Luque J et al. Chemotherapy-induced eccrine squamous syringometaplasia. *Arch Dermatol* 1997; 133: 873–8.

See also case number 34.

Case 9
Painful pustules in pregnancy

History

A 16-year-old girl presented at 31 weeks gestation with a 4-week history of a pustular eruption that developed initially on the periumbilical skin. Subsequently the eruption spread to involve the breasts, back, flexures and proximal limbs. The dermatosis was associated with cutaneous pain, fever and malaise. This was her second pregnancy, the first being terminated at 12 weeks. The patient had no past history of skin disease and had not developed a rash during her previous pregnancy.

Clinical findings

The patient was febrile (38.7°C) and appeared ill. On the trunk there were sharply demarcated, erythematous plaques studded with pustules (Figure 9a). On the periumbilical skin the pustules were arranged in concentric rings (Figure 9b) while on the breasts there was coalescence of pustules forming lakes of pus. The patient was tachycardic but haemodynamically stable. Fetal movements were frequent.

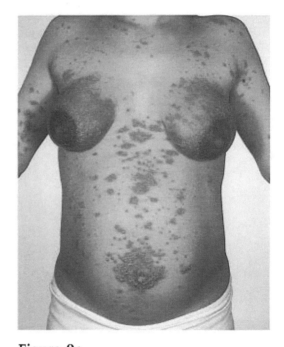

Figure 9a

Generalized pustular psoriasis of pregnancy.
There are multiple inflamed pustular plaques on the trunk with predilection for the breasts and periumbilical skin.

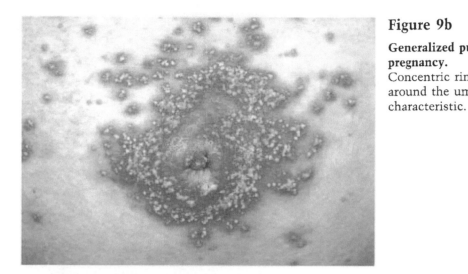

Figure 9b

Generalized pustular psoriasis of pregnancy.
Concentric rings of small pustules around the umbilicus are characteristic.

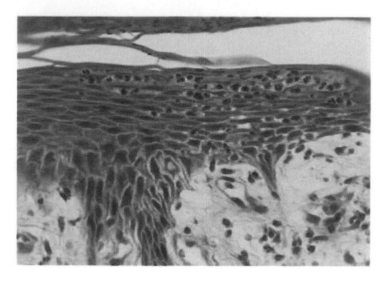

Figure 9c

Generalized pustular psoriasis of pregnancy.
Skin histopathology (H&E, high power). There is a subcorneal, spongiotic pustule (of Kogoj) containing neutrophils. Sterile subcorneal pustules are characteristic of active pustular psoriasis.

Investigations

Hb: 10.5 g/dl (11.5–15.5 g/dl), WCC: 14.6 × 10^9/l (4.0–11.0 × 10^9/l), PMN: 12.4 × 10^9/l (2.0–5.0 × 10^9/l), plts: 263 × 10^9/l (150–450 × 10^9/l). ESR: 43 mm/hr (1–10 mm/hr).

U&E: normal, LFT: normal, albumin: 20 g/l (35–50 g/l), corrected calcium: 2.02 mmol/l (2.2–2.4 mmol/l).

Skin swabs: negative bacterial culture.

Blood culture: negative.

Skin histopathology: Biopsy of periumbilical skin demonstrated psoriasiform acanthosis with subcorneal, spongiform neutrophil-rich pustules. There was overlying parakeratosis (Figure 9c).

Diagnosis

Generalized pustular psoriasis of pregnancy.

Treatment and progress

The patient was admitted and initially treated conservatively with bed rest and emollients. However, with extension of the eruption and persistent fever, pulsed intramuscular dexamethasone was given on 2 consecutive days, followed by prednisolone 60 mg daily. Despite high-dose corticosteroid the pustulation increased to involve 80% of the body surface area and was associated with decreased fetal movements. A decision was made to deliver the fetus and a female infant was born via Caesarean section 10 days after the patient's admission (33 weeks gestation). At 12 hours of age the baby developed a tension pneumothorax, which was drained. In the following days the infant became increasingly unwell and died of a pulmonary haemorrhage at 9 days of age.

Following the Caesarean section the mother's pustulation failed to improve and so treatment with methotrexate was initiated, which controlled the eruption. Two months later the methotrexate was discontinued without relapse.

Four years later the patient re-presented to the dermatology department, 11 weeks pregnant. She first suspected that she may be pregnant following the development of pustules around the umbilicus. The pregnancy was terminated 1 week later but the eruption persisted after the termination and, on this occasion, required a 2-month course of cyclosporin to induce a remission.

Comment

A widespread pustular eruption occurring in pregnancy, as characterized by this patient, was originally called 'impetigo herpetiformis', but is now generally regarded as generalized pustular psoriasis (GPP) of pregnancy. The eruption usually develops in the third trimester and characteristically initially involves the flexures and periumbilical skin. Small sterile pustules appear on areas of acutely inflamed skin that subsequently expand. The pattern of concentric rings of pustules developing around the umbilicus, as seen in our patient, has been observed in other reported cases. Severe constitutional upset is common in GPP of pregnancy, with fever, arthralgia and gastrointestinal symptoms being frequently reported. Blood tests demonstrate hypoalbuminaemia and hypocalcaemia. The condition tends to persist until delivery and carries an associated mortality from cardiac or renal failure.

The main obstetric problem is placental insufficiency with an increased risk of still-birth, neonatal death and fetal abnormalities. The disease characteristically recurs with each pregnancy, with earlier onset and increased morbidity. Between pregnancies, patients are generally free of the disorder and have no manifestations of psoriasis.

Pustulation in GPP of psoriasis is difficult to control. Corticosteroids have been used in many cases with varying success while more recent reports have identified cyclosporin as a beneficial agent without appreciable fetal morbidity. In some cases the only effective treatment is termination of the pregnancy. In other cases continued post-partum pustulation requires systemic therapy to control cutaneous inflammation.

Learning points

1. Pregnancy can be associated with an aggressive form of acute generalized pustular psoriasis.
2. The condition is associated with considerable morbidity and mortality to both mother and fetus.
3. Systemic therapy is usually required. However, severe cases may only respond to termination of the pregnancy.

Reference

Breier-Maly J, Ortel B, Breier F et al. Generalized pustular psoriasis of pregnancy. *Dermatology* 1999; 198: 61–4.

See also case number 22.

Case 10
Discharging nodules on the jaw

History

A 46-year-old Jamaican man presented with an 8-month history of painful swellings over the left side of his jaw. The patient was unable to open his mouth fully and had noticed that the swollen areas sometimes discharged pus. The patient had a past history of scarring acne but was otherwise well. Before being referred to the dermatology department he had been seen by his dentist, who had noted multiple caries.

Clinical findings

On examination, there were three hard, indurated, fixed swellings over the left side of the jaw (Figure 10a). Two of these were discharging pus to the skin surface (Figure 10b). The surrounding skin was firm and tethered. There was no regional lymphadenopathy. The right side of the jaw was normal. Inspection of the oral cavity revealed very poor dentition.

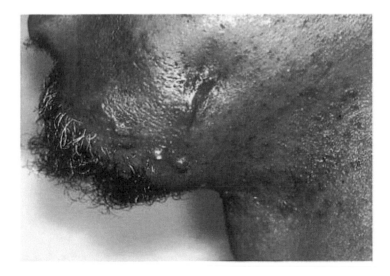

Figure 10a

Cervicofacial actinomycosis.
There are nodules and scarring over the left side of the jaw.

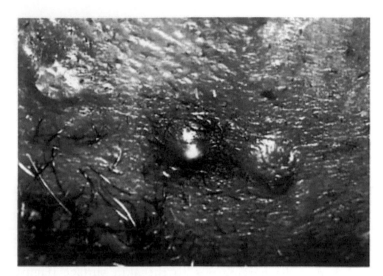

Figure 10b

Cervicofacial actinomycosis.
The central lesion was a discharging sinus. The presence of sinuses helps to distinguish this condition from nodulocystic acne.

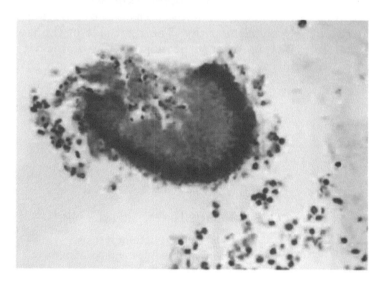

Figure 10c

Cervicofacial actinomycosis.
Histopathology from a deep biopsy of the subcutaneous tissue (H&E, high power). There is a 'sulphur' granule with a filamentous edge. Granules represent dense aggregates of *Actinomyces* filaments.

Investigations

Microscopy of pus smear: 'sulphur' granules.

Skin histopathology: A deep biopsy of the skin of the jaw revealed fibrosis of the mid and deep dermis and, at the deep margins, numerous 'sulphur' granules (Figure 10c).

Chest x-ray: normal.

MRI jaw: There was severe periodontal disease with overlying soft tissue inflammation.

Diagnosis

Cervicofacial actinomycosis.

Treatment and progress

The patient was given a 3-month course of penicillin V, 250 mg four times a day. After 2 months there was clearance of the infection with no further purulent discharge. By completion of treatment the sinuses were healed and the sclerotic areas were showing signs of resolution.

Comment

Actinomyces israelii is a Gram-positive anaerobic bacillus that is part of a heterogenous group related to mycobacteria but resembling fungi. They are filamentous and branching and form thin-walled, asexual spores. *A. israelii* is a normal oral commensal organism which may become pathogenic following trauma to the jaw or, as in our case, as a result of periodontal disease. Lesions start as painless swellings and harden to woody nodules (hence the terms 'woody jaw' or 'lumpy jaw'), which then break down, suppurate and form sinus tracts that open externally. These foci infect surrounding tissues so that simultaneous healing with scar formation in one area and new sinus formation in contiguous areas is characteristic. A number of cases of cervicofacial actinomycosis are accompanied by chest involvement, which may be caused by direct spread from buccal infection.

Actinomycosis is characterized by the presence of 'sulphur' granules seen on microscopy of a smear of the pus. These granules are actually dense meshes of *Actinomyces* filaments that become lobulated. *A. israelii* can be cultured under anaerobic conditions to yield creamy-white colonies. Since *A. israelii* is very slowly growing, treatment with long courses of antibiotics is necessary. The organism is usually sensitive to penicillins, but other options include erythromycin, tetracycline, rifampicin and chloramphenicol. Surgical treatment is sometimes required if the response to antibiotics is poor.

> ## Learning points
>
> 1. Localized nodular induration of the skin of the jaw should suggest a diagnosis of cervicofacial actinomycosis.
> 2. Cervicofacial actinomycosis results from local, soft-tissue spread of oral *Actinomyces*, usually as a consequence of periodontal disease or trauma to the mandible.
> 3. 'Sulphur' granules, which are aggregates of *Actinomyces* organisms, can be seen microscopically in pus expressed from a purulent lesion or in tissue from a deep, surgical biopsy.

Reference

Lerner PI. The lumpy jaw. Cervicofacial actinomycosis. *Infect Dis Clin North Am* 1988; 2: 203–20.

See also case number 24.

Case 11
Thickening of the facial skin, weakness of the hands and loss of peripheral sensation

History

A 53-year-old Anglo-Indian man presented with a 3-year history of thickening of his facial skin with the development of numerous papules and nodules. He also complained of weakness of the right hand and altered sensation in the fingers of both hands and numbness of his feet. The patient had emigrated to the United Kingdom from India 5 years previously.

Clinical findings

Examination of the face revealed thickened skin of the forehead, nose and cheeks. There were deep, longitudinal furrows in the skin of the forehead and numerous indurated nodules involving the nose, lips and ears (Figures 11a, b). Examination of the hands showed dystrophy of the nails of the right hand, ulnar deviation of the right little finger and wasting of the first dorsal interosseus muscles (Figure 11c).

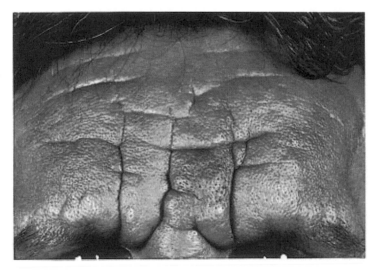

Figure 11a

Lepromatous leprosy.
Thickened skin of the forehead with deep longitudinal furrows and prominent transverse creases producing the so-called 'leonine' facies.

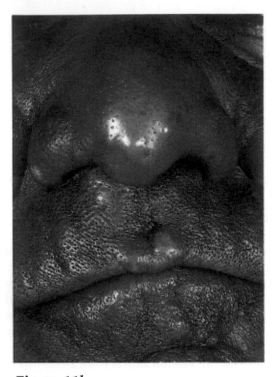

Figure 11b

Lepromatous leprosy.
There are dermal nodules on the nose and lips. Acral sites, such as these, are characteristically involved in lepromatous leprosy.

There was widespread skin dryness (Figure 11d). Neurological examination demonstrated a right-sided ulnar nerve palsy and evidence of bilateral peripheral sensory loss in a glove-and-stocking distribution. He had multiple thickened nerves (right and left ulnar, left median, right and left radial and ulnar cutaneous nerves).

Investigations

Skin histopathology: Biopsies taken from the skin of the eyebrow and ear showed sheets of pale staining macrophages with foamy cytoplasm, in places forming whorls around peripheral nerves. Wade–Fite stain revealed innumerable acid-fast bacilli within the macrophages (Figure 11e).

Diagnosis

Lepromatous leprosy.

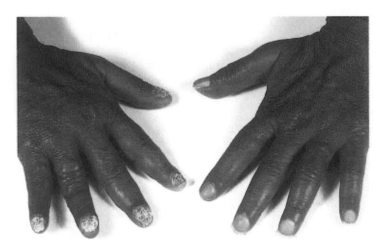

Figure 11c

Lepromatous leprosy.
Fusiform changes of the fingers of both hands with wasting of the first dorsal interosseous muscles. There is ulnar deviation of the right little finger secondary to lepromatous bone involvement. There is also a tinea infection of the nails of the right hand.

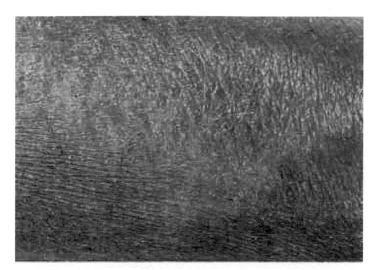

Figure 11d

Lepromatous leprosy.
There is widespread dryness of the skin in lepromatous disease, as demonstrated in this picture of the patient's arm.

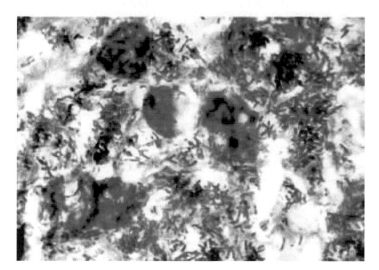

Figure 11e

Lepromatous leprosy.
Skin biopsy from nodule on the ear (Wade–Fite stain, high power), showing macrophages with numerous *M. leprae* bacilli within the cytoplasm.

Treatment and progress

The patient was treated for 2 years with the World Health Organization (WHO) recommended multidrug therapy regimen: rifampicin and clofazimine monthly and dapsone daily. Towards the end of this treatment he developed erythema nodosum leprosum, which required treatment with prednisolone and thalidomide. Despite physiotherapy and orthotic foot care he developed recurrent neuropathic foot ulcers and required multiple orthopaedic interventions.

Although the patient felt strongly stigmatized by the diagnosis of leprosy, he lived for a further 15 years after the diagnosis was made and died from an unrelated illness.

Comment

Leprosy is caused by *Mycobacterium leprae* infection, which induces a chronic inflammatory disease primarily involving the skin and nerves. *M. leprae* is of low infectivity and prolonged contact with an affected individual is necessary for transmission. The subsequent incubation period lasts several years. Leprosy occurs most commonly in developing countries of the tropics and subtropics.

The clinical manifestations of leprosy reflect the host's immune response to *M. leprae*. In lepromatous leprosy failure of cell-mediated immunity leads to bacillary multiplication and haematogenous spread of bacilli to cool superficial sites, including the acral tissues of the face, hands and feet. Early involvement of the nasal mucosa in lepromatous disease results in nasal stuffiness and discharge while involvement of the skin produces skin-coloured papules and nodules on the face and limbs. With time, the facial skin thickens, the forehead creases deepen, eyebrows are lost and the nose broadens producing the typical 'leonine' facies. Slow fibrosis of peripheral nerves results in bilateral glove-and-stocking anaesthesia. However, in contrast with a typical polyneuropathy, sensation on the palms and soles is spared, as are the deep tendon reflexes, until late in the disease course. As the disease progresses the peripheral nerves become at first firm and then enlarged. In lepromatous leprosy the hands and feet take on a characteristic appearance with swollen, fusiform digits with tapering ends. Lepromatous inflammation in the small bones of the hands leads to osteopenia and pathological fractures that, as in our patient, tend to heal with misalignment.

Patients with multibacillary leprosy should be treated with a triple-drug regimen of rifampicin, dapsone and clofazimine for 24 months. Treatment complication with erythma nodosum leprosum (ENL), as seen in our case, occurs in one half of patients and represents an immunological reaction (type 2) to a large load of dead bacilli. ENL manifests as painful red nodules on the face and extensor surfaces of the limbs accompanied by fever, malaise, arthritis, myositis, neuritis and uveitis.

Most of the disability in leprosy results from loss of sensation due to neuropathy. Once *M. leprae* infection has been eradicated long-term management should be directed at limiting traumatic and orthopaedic complications from nerve damage.

Learning points

1. Leprosy should be considered in a patient from an endemic area who presents with skin lesions and peripheral nerve abnormalities.
2. Lepromatous leprosy presents with multiple papules and nodules distributed bilaterally and symmetrically, usually involving the facial skin.
3. The diagnosis of lepromatous leprosy is made by identifying numerous lepromatous bacilli in the skin biopsy.

Reference

Sasaki S, Takeshita F, Okuda K, Ishii N. *Mycobacterium leprae* and leprosy. *Microbiol Immunol* 2001; 45: 729–36.

See also case number 39.

Case 12
A facial and anogenital rash in an infant

History

A 6-month-old baby boy presented with a 1-week history of an eruption involving, predominantly, the facial and anogenital skin. The patient had been born at term and was well during the first 6 months of life. The onset of the eruption coincided with weaning from breast milk to cow's milk. There was no relevant family history.

Clinical findings

On examination, there were well-demarcated, glazed, erythematous lesions around the mouth, eyes, the nappy area and the knees (Figures 12a, b). There was confluent involvement of the perianal skin, inner thighs and scrotum, which, in places, was eroded and exudative. There was oral candidiasis.

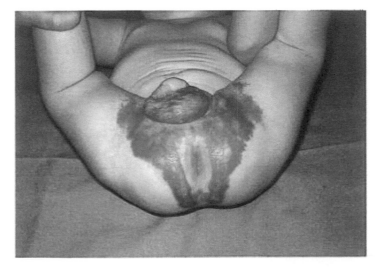

Figure 12a

Acrodermatitis enteropathica.
On presentation at 6 months of age, there was well-demarcated, glazed erythema involving scrotal, groin and perianal skin.

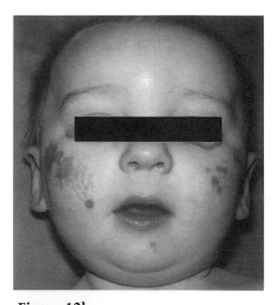

Figure 12b

Acrodermatitis enteropathica.
The eruption on the face was less marked than
the anogenital involvement. There were patches
of erythema around the eyes and on the cheeks.

Investigations

Serum zinc: 3.2 µmol/l (10.1–29.7 µmol/l).

Diagnosis

Acrodermatitis enteropathica.

Treatment and progress

The patient was commenced on oral zinc 50
mg/day. Breast feeding was reintroduced. His
rash resolved rapidly and was completely
clear 4 weeks after initiation of zinc supplementation (Figure 12c). Over the ensuing 12
months his zinc requirements required to
control the eruption increased from 50 mg to
300 mg per day. Two years after presentation
the patient's rash reappeared and was associated with diarrhoea. The serum zinc level
was again found to be low and oral supplementation was increased further. He has
since remained well.

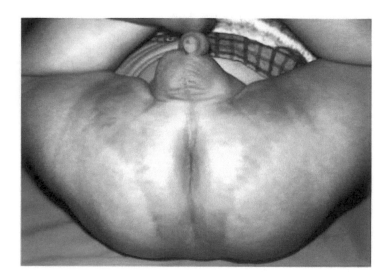

Figure 12c

Acrodermatitis enteropathica.
After 3 weeks of zinc replacement
clearance of the eruption was
virtually complete.

Comment

Acrodermatitis enteropathica (AE) is a rare autosomal recessive nutritional deficiency disorder resulting from defective intestinal absorption of zinc. In 1973 Moynahan and Barnes first identified the clinical association with zinc while studying a patient with AE and associated lactose intolerance. They observed that alterations in zinc concentrations affected the well-being of the patient, leading to the discovery that AE was a disease of zinc deficiency. Prior to this finding, the disease was usually fatal in infancy or childhood but is now rapidly and dramatically cured by dietary supplementation with zinc salts.

In affected infants who are bottle-fed with cow's milk AE usually begins within days to a few weeks after birth. In breast-fed children the disease begins soon after weaning. The clinical onset is characterized by scaly, eczematous plaques on the face, anogenital areas and scalp, where it is associated with alopecia. The hands and feet are also commonly involved, with paronychia and a dermatitis of the palmar and finger creases. Without zinc replacement, lesions may become vesicobullous or pustular and, as the dermatitis worsens, secondary infections with bacteria and *Candida albicans* can occur. Diarrhoea is the most variable manifestation of AE and may be only intermittent, as in our patient, or totally absent. If AE is left untreated, growth failure becomes measurable within weeks and clinically apparent as the child approaches adolescence. In boys with untreated AE, hypogonadism becomes evident at puberty.

Learning points

1. Acrodermatitis enteropathica (AE) should be considered in an infant with a facial and anogenital dermatosis developing shortly after weaning from breast to cow's milk.
2. AE is a genetically determined defect in intestinal absorption of zinc.
3. Extracutaneous manifestations of AE include diarrhoea, growth failure and, if untreated, hypogonadism in males.

The identification of zinc malabsorption as the critical defect in AE has provoked interest in the mechanism of zinc transport in the gut. The fact that zinc in human milk is considerably more biologically available to infants with AE than zinc from cow's milk suggests the involvement of a species-specific zinc-binding ligand. Recent mutational analysis studies have identified a candidate gene in AE families that encodes a protein with features of a zinc-specific transporter.

Reference

Kury S, Dreno B, Bezieau S et al. Identification of *SLC39A4*, a gene involved in acrodermatitis enteropathica. *Nat Genet* 2002; 31: 239–40.

See also case number 31.

Case 13
Non-healing dog bites

History

A 68-year old man was admitted 5 days after sustaining three dog bites. Examination revealed two painful and necrotic wounds on the left thigh and one on the right thigh. Surrounding each lesion was a zone of erythema. He was commenced on intravenous antibiotics and taken to the operating theatre for excision of necrotic tissue. Two days later he underwent further surgical debridement of new necrotic tissue, including underlying muscle; 48 hours later he was still febrile with continued expansion of the wounds. During this period he was noted to develop inflammatory and necrotic areas at the sites of venous canulation. The antibiotic regime was changed and further debridement was proposed. Whilst the patient was being prepared for surgery, a dermatology opinion was requested.

Clinical findings

On examination, he was found to have eight lesions with dark margins: three at the sites of the original dog bites and five others at sites of venous cannulation, venepuncture and arterial blood sampling (Figure 13a). The leg lesions were ulcerated with dusky margins. The lesions of the arms were superficial and erythematous with a blistering margin (Figure 13b).

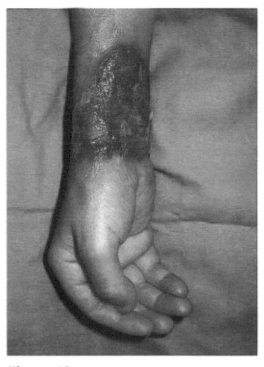

Figure 13a

Pyoderma gangrenosum.
A superficial lesion at the right wrist that developed at the site of arterial blood sampling.

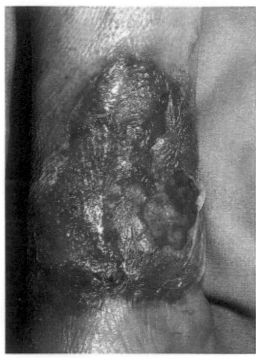

Figure 13b

Pyoderma gangrenosum.
A closer view of the lesion in Figure 13a
demonstrates the inflammatory, blistering
margin.

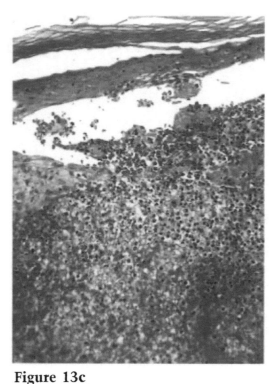

Figure 13c

Pyoderma gangrenosum.
Skin histopathology from right wrist
lesion (H&E, medium power). There is
sub-epidermal blister formation with a
dense collection of neutrophils in the
dermis, resembling an abscess.

Investigations

Hb: 9.4 g/dl (11.5–15.5 g/dl), WCC: 19.7 ×
10^9/l (4.0–11.0 × 10^9/l), PMN: 14.4 × 10^9/l
(2.0–5.0 × 10^9/l), plts: 458 × 10^9/l (150–450 ×
10^9/l). ESR: 67 mm/hr (1–10 mm/hr).

Blood culture: negative.

Tissue culture: negative.

Skin histopathology: Biopsy of the edge of an
arm lesion demonstrated blistering with a
dense, neutrophilic cellular infiltrate throughout the underlying dermis (Figure 13c).

Diagnosis

Pyoderma gangrenosum.

Treatment and progress

The patient was immediately commenced on
prednisolone 80 mg once daily. There was a
dramatic improvement in his clinical condition, with rapid resolution of fever and

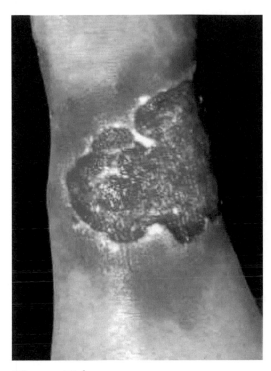

Figure 13d

Pyoderma gangrenosum.
A few days after commencing high dose
oral corticosteroid the dusky margins
surrounding the lesions settled and
grannulation tissue developed at the base
of the ulcers.

clearance of perilesional erythema (Figure
13d). Re-epithelialization of the ulcers
commenced a few days later. The patient
was investigated for underlying gastrointestinal, rheumatological and haematological
disease; all investigations were negative.
Over the ensuing 6 months the dose of
systemic corticosteroid was gradually
reduced and ultimately discontinued without
relapse of the pyoderma gangrenosum.

Comment

Pyoderma gangrenosum (PG) is a destructive
skin disorder presenting usually as a painful
ulcer with necrotic, undermined margins.
Lesions may develop either in isolation or, in
50% of cases, in association with systemic
disease, most commonly inflammatory
bowel disease, rheumatoid arthritis or
haematological malignancy (most commonly
acute or chronic myeloid leukaemia and
multiple myeloma). As well as an ulcerative
form, a number of other clinical subtypes of
PG have been characterized, including
bullous, pustular and superficial granulomatous variants. In our patient the leg lesions
were typical of ulcerative PG while the arm
lesions were superficial and inflammatory.

Provocation of PG lesions by trauma is
termed 'pathergy' and is observed in approximately 20% of cases. Our patient had a
strongly pathergic response with lesions
being triggered by the initial dog bites, the
debriding surgery, venepuncture and venous
cannulation. This phenomenon indicates an
uncontrolled wounding response in which
local factors interact with tissue damage to
provoke an intense neutrophilic inflammatory response. Pathergy is also observed in
other dermatoses that share a neutrophilic
tissue reaction, including Sweet's syndrome
and Behçet's disease.

The pathogenesis of the neutrophilic
dermatoses remains obscure. Inflammatory
cytokines and neutrophil chemoattractant
factors appear to be important in generating
a neutrophil-rich dermal infiltrate. The
ulcer formation in PG may be induced by
destructive factors generated by activated
neutrophils, such as peroxidase and reactive
oxygen species.

Once diagnosed, the initial management of
PG should be directed to a search for a possible associated systemic disease and, there-

Learning points

1. Pyoderma gangrenosum (PG) commonly presents as a rapidly expanding ulcer with dark undermined margins. Other variants include bullous, pustular and superficial granulomatous forms.
2. PG may demonstrate pathergy, defined as the provocation of the disease at a site of skin piercing or cutting.
3. 50% of cases are associated with an underlying disease, most commonly inflammatory bowel disease, rheumatoid arthritis or haematological malignancy.

after, its treatment. The most consistently successful agent in the therapy of PG is high-dose corticosteroid, either oral prednisolone or pulsed intravenous methylprednisolone. Other drugs used successfully, often in combination with corticosteroids, include dapsone, clofazimine and cyclosporin.

Reference

Powell FC, Su WPD, Perry HO. Pyoderma gangrenosum: classification and management. *J Am Acad Dermatol* 1996; 34: 395–409.

See also case number 20.

Case 14
Two patients with pustular plaques on a neurosurgical ward

History

A 43-year-old woman was admitted following a fall from a second-storey window. She had sustained a contusion of the spinal cord resulting in tetraplegia. This patient received high-dose dexamethasone and was nursed on a spinal injuries bed. A rash was noted on her back 10 days after admission.

Two weeks later a second patient on the same ward developed a similar eruption. This patient was a 33-year-old man, who had sustained a whiplash injury that resulted in tetraplegia. He was admitted to the neurosurgical unit, where he was also treated with high-dose dexamethasone and was nursed on an identical spinal injuries bed. Twelve days after admission the nurses noticed a rash on his back.

Clinical findings

Both patients had a similar eruption characterized by several well-circumscribed, erythematous plaques on the skin of the back (Figures 14a, b). The surfaces of these lesions were studded with superficial pustules (Figure 14c).

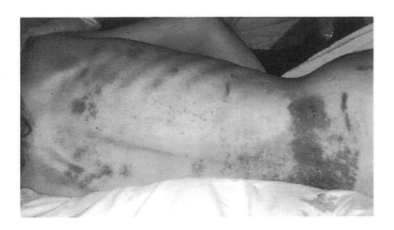

Figure 14a

Primary cutaneous aspergillosis.
Case 1. Multiple erythematous lesions were found on the back of this tetraplegic patient nursed on a spinal injuries bed.

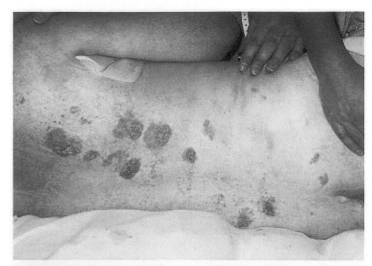

Figure 14b

Primary cutaneous aspergillosis.
Case 2. A second patient on the neurosurgical unit developed a similar eruption of pustular plaques on his back.

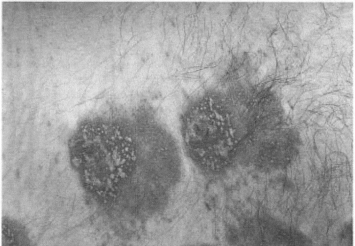

Figure 14c

Primary cutaneous aspergillosis.
The lesions in both patients consisted of small superficial pustules on an erythematosus base.

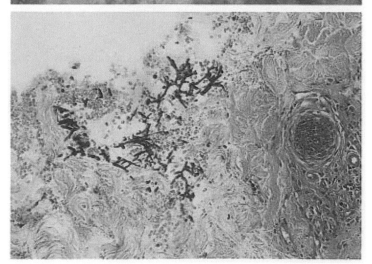

Figure 14d

Primary cutaneous aspergillosis.
Skin histopathology (PAS, medium power). There are septate, dichotomously branching fungi in the dermis.

Investigations

Skin histopathology: Biopsies from both patients revealed septate, dichotomously branching fungi present in the dermis (Figure 14d).

Culture of skin biopsy: *Aspergillus fumigatus* was grown from both biopsies.

Cultures from blood, urine, sputum and bronchoalveolar lavage: negative.

Serum aspergillus precipitins: negative.

Diagnosis

Primary cutaneous aspergillosis.

Treatment and progress

Both cases responded completely to a 2-week course of itraconazole 200 mg twice daily. Further investigations to identify the source of infection demonstrated a positive *Aspergillus* culture from the bed sheets in the second case and also from the air vent supplying the ward. Building works were taking place in the grounds of the hospital close to the neurosurgical unit.

Comment

Aspergillus spp. are ubiquitous organisms and represent the second most common cause of opportunistic fungal infection, surpassed only by *Candida* spp. Under normal conditions, an intact skin and functioning immune system provide an effective barrier against colonization by *Aspergillus* spp. However, serious infection can occur in immunocompromised subjects exposed to air containing numerous *Aspergillus* spores released from nearby construction sites.

Primary cutaneous aspergillosis requires direct inoculation of the fungus into the skin from the external environment and is most commonly reported in neutropenic patients, but has also been recorded in patients receiving immunosuppressant drugs, in HIV-positive individuals and in neonates. Both of our patients received dexamethasone as a part of their neurosurgical treatment, inducing a degree of immunosuppression and encouraging the inoculated spores to germinate. Immobility will have resulted in prolonged skin contact with contaminated bed linen, further encouraging invasion by *Aspergillus*.

The morphological characteristics of primary cutaneous aspergillosis are variable; pustules, vesiculopustular plaques, nodules and ulcers have all been described. Since the clinical appearances may mimic other

---

Learning points

1. Aspergillosis should be considered in the differential diagnosis of a pustular eruption occurring in an immunocompromised patient.
2. Although *Aspergillus spp.* can be cultured from a skin swab, the diagnosis should be made by taking a skin biopsy for histopathology and fungal culture.
3. Hospital-acquired infection may occur via air contaminated with *Aspergillus* spores that have been released from nearby building works.

dermatoses, skin swabs for culture and a skin biopsy for histology and culture are recommended in suspected cases. Once primary cutaneous aspergillosis is diagnosed treatment should be directed to local measures and systemic anti-fungal therapy. Local treatment includes excision of infected skin, especially if the lesions are deep-seated. Itraconazole is preferred in non-neutropenic immunocompromised subjects, such as our cases, while amphotericin B therapy is most appropriate for neonates and patients with neutropenia. The majority of cases resolve with appropriate therapy. However, a propor-

tion may proceed to systemic aspergillosis, which carries a significant mortality.

Reference

Van Burik J-AH, Colven R, Spach DH. Cutaneous aspergillosis. *J Clin Microbiol* 1998; 36: 3115–21.

See also case number 33.

Case 15
Fever and purpuric lesions in an infant

History

A 14-month-old baby boy presented with a 2-day history of a fever and skin lesions. In the 6 days prior to this he had developed a cough and was noted to be lethargic. The general practitioner had commenced the child on erythromycin without benefit. There was no past medical history of note.

Clinical findings

The infant looked ill and was febrile (39.2°C). Examination of the skin revealed multiple, urticated, purpuric lesions distributed mainly on his face, hands and feet (Figures 15a, b). These were 1–2 cm in diameter, round with a well-defined margin (Figure 15c). Oedema was noted on the eyelids and on the flexor surfaces of the hands and feet.

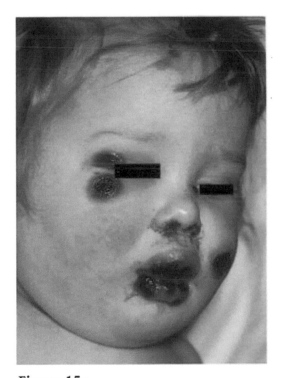

Figure 15a

Acute haemorrhagic oedema of infancy. Oedematous, discoid, purpuric lesions are present on the cheeks and eyelids. There is also involvement of the lips and nostrils.

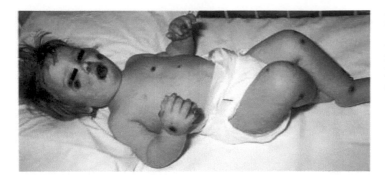

Figure 15b

Acute haemorrhagic oedema of infancy.
Lesions are distributed predominantly on the face, hands and legs.

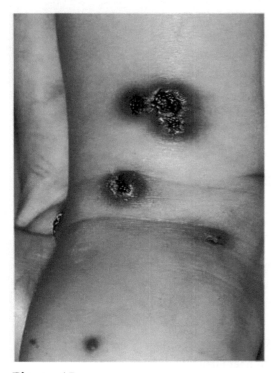

Figure 15c

Acute haemorrhagic oedema of infancy.
Multiple raised necrotic and haemorrhagic lesions are present on the left lower leg and dorsum of the foot.

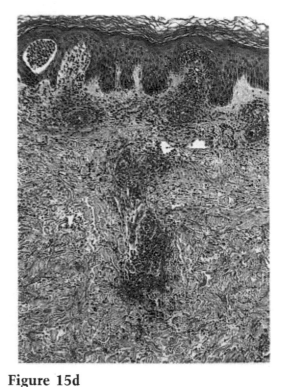

Figure 15d

Acute haemorrhagic oedema of infancy.
Skin histopathology (H&E, low power). There is leucocytoclastic vasculitis with a neutrophil-rich perivascular infiltrate, endothelial cell swelling, fibrinoid necrosis of vessel walls and extravasated erythrocytes.

Investigations

Hb: 10.7 g/dl (11.5–15.5 g/dl), WCC: 19 × 10^9/l (4.0–11.0 × 10^9/l), PMN: 11.0 × 10^9/l (2.0–5.0 × 10^9/l), lymphs, 6.9 × 10^9/l (1.0–3.0 × 10^9/l), plts: 567 × 10^9/l (150–450 × 10^9/l). ESR: 39 mm/hr (1–10 mm/hr).

U&E: normal, LFT: normal, autoantibodies: normal.

Blood cultures: negative, lumbar puncture: normal, MSU: negative, throat swab: normal, skin swab: negative.

Skin histopathology: Biopsy revealed a small-vessel leucocytoclastic vasculitis with fibrinoid necrosis involving the vessels of the upper and mid dermis (Figure 15d).

Adenovirus serology: IgM-positive.

Diagnosis

Acute haemorrhagic oedema of the skin in infancy.

Treatment and progress

Once an infective process had been excluded the patient was commenced on prednisolone 3 mg/kg/day, which resulted in an immediate resolution of the fever and a rapid clearance of the skin lesions. The corticosteroids were reduced as the eruption settled, and 2 weeks after admission prednisolone was discontinued altogether. He remained well on discharge and had no recurrence of the dermatosis.

Comment

Acute haemorrhagic oedema of the skin in infancy (AHOI) is a rare cutaneous disease that almost exclusively affects children under 2 years of age. The presentation of the eruption is acute but the evolution of the disorder is generally benign, with spontaneous resolution often occurring within a few weeks. The differential diagnosis of AHOI includes the necrotic purpura of meningococcaemia, Henoch–Schönlein purpura (HSP), urticarial vasculitis, erythema multiforme and Sweet's syndrome. Clinically and pathologically, AHOI is most closely related to HSP and overlap forms between these two disorders exist. AHOI is characterized by oedematous purpuric lesions, typically *en cocarde* in appearance (rosette-like) and localized predominantly on the face (cheeks, eyelids and ears) and limbs (mainly the extremities). Systemic involvement is rare. In contrast, HSP is typified by palpable purpura predominantly involving the lower legs and occurring in association with variable involvement of the gastrointestinal tract, joints and kidneys. The histological

---

Learning points

1. In a child presenting with purpuric or necrotic skin lesions meningococcal septicaemia must be excluded as a priority.
2. Clinically, AHOI is characterized by oedematous discoid purpuric lesions with predilection for the face, hands, legs and feet.
3. Generally, AHOI runs a benign course without systemic involvement.

pattern of leucocytoclastic vasculitis is similar in AHOI and HSP; however, immunofluorescence studies have reported the preponderance of vascular C1q deposition in AHOI, in contrast to IgA and C3 in HSP.

In the limited literature on the subject spontaneous and complete resolution of AHOI occurs within 1–3 weeks and the disease is generally considered to run a benign course. Many reported cases have resolved without the need for systemic medication. However, the severity of involvement in our case necessitated the use of prednisolone. Although the origin of AHOI is not clear, a history of infection is elicited in 75% of cases and in our case serological tests clearly demonstrated a primary infection with adenovirus. It has been suggested that in AHOI the host immune response to cells expressing viral antigen may be the stimulus for cutaneous vasculitis.

Reference

Legrain V, Lejean S, Taieb A et al. Infantile acute hemorrhagic oedema of the skin: study of ten cases. *J Am Acad Dermatol* 1991; 24: 17–22.

See also case numbers 43, 50.

Case 16
Photosensitivity with skin cancers

History

A 2-year-old girl presented with a history of photosensitivity and the appearance of unusual freckling on her facial skin. She was born of healthy, unrelated parents and had an unaffected non-identical twin sister. Her parents had noticed that, since birth, she displayed a very florid sunburn reaction to minimal summer sunlight exposure with, on occasions, blistering of affected skin. She was noted to be photophobic and actively avoided sunlight. At an early age she developed keratotic lesions on the skin of her face and by the age of 10 several tumours (basal cell and squamous cell carcinomas) had been excised from the skin of her face and arms (Figure 16a). During her early teens she was also noted to have developed bilateral perceptive deafness. At the age of 12 she presented with a large, rapidly growing tumour arising from the skin of the nasal tip (Figure 16b).

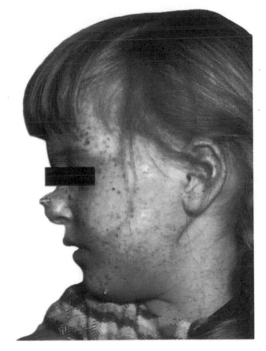

Figure 16a

Xeroderma pigmentosum.
The patient aged 6 years. There are numerous freckles and a keratotic lesion on the nose. Excision demonstrated a squamous cell carcinoma.

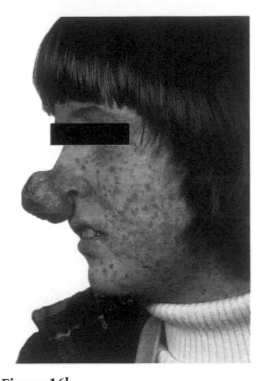 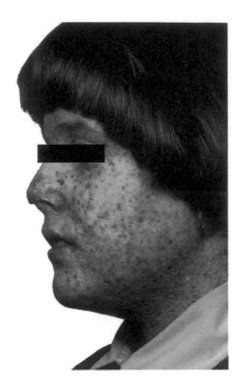

Figure 16b

Kerato-acanthoma and xeroderma pigmentosum.
Left: The patient aged 12 years. A 4 cm diameter kerato-acanthoma has developed on the nasal tip. *Right:* Six months later the kerato-acanthoma underwent complete self-healing.

Clinical findings

Examination of the exposed skin of the face and hands demonstrated extensive freckling with numerous large tan-coloured lentigines, interspersed with areas of pallor (Figure 16c). The skin was generally dry. There was evidence of bilateral keratitis with early pterygium formation of the right eye. A 4 cm diameter firm nodule replaced the skin of the nasal tip. The tumour was dome-shaped with a keratotic apex.

Investigations

Skin histopathology: biopsy of the tumour revealed a well-differentiated squamous cell carcinoma, with architecture consistent with a kerato-acanthoma.

DNA repair studies performed on the patient's cultured fibroblasts demonstrated a marked reduction in unscheduled DNA synthesis, consistent with xeroderma pigmentosum (XP). Complementation studies assigned her to XP group A.

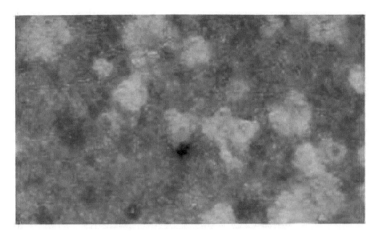

Figure 16c

Xeroderma pigmentosum.
The skin displays the signs of severe photodamage with lentigines of varying size and pigmentation interspersed with areas of hypopigmentation.

Diagnosis

Xeroderma pigmentosum, group A.

Treatment and progress

The large kerato-acanthoma involving the nasal tip underwent spontaneous resolution leaving minor scarring. Despite scrupulous avoidance of sunlight and use of high-protection-factor sunscreens, the patient continued to develop numerous actinic keratoses and skin cancers. By the age of 25 she had undergone the excision of more than 100 tumours (BCC:SCC ratio approximately 5:1). At the age of 35 years she developed a lentigo maligna melanoma on the left leg.

Psychological problems developed during childhood, resulting in anxiety and depression. She became socially withdrawn and reclusive. Progressive neurological complications resulted in cerebellar limb ataxia, ataxic dysarthria and oropharyngeal dysphagia. At the age of 30 an MRI of the head demonstrated that the brain and brainstem

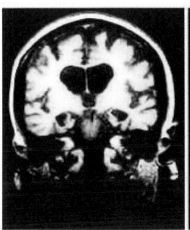
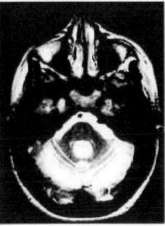

Figure 16d

Xeroderma pigmentosum, complementation group A.
In complementation group A there is an associated degenerative neurological disorder. MRI of the head: *left:* Coronal T1-weighted image through the cerebrum showing expanded ventricles and widening cerebral sulci. *Right:* Axial T2-weighted image through the cerebellum showing enlarged fourth ventricle and widened cerebellar fissures.

were small. There were atrophic changes with widening of the lateral, third and fourth ventricles. There was a widening of the cortical sulci and of the spaces between cerebral folia (Figure 16d). By the age of 35, her neurological disabilities had rendered her deaf, partially sighted, unable to stand unaided and entirely dependent on the care of her mother.

Comment

Xeroderma pigmentosum (XP) is an autosomal recessive genetic defect of the DNA repair mechanism. Under normal circumstances, UV-damaged DNA in the skin is removed from the genome and replaced by new intact DNA by nucleotide excision repair (NER), a multi-step process involving several enzymes and cofactors. If left untreated, UV-induced DNA lesions (photoadducts) interfere with normal DNA function and can ultimately produce mutations. Consequently, defective NER in XP permits unchecked progression of genomic UV damage in skin, resulting in accelerated photoageing and photocarcinogenesis.

XP presents in infancy with an exaggerated sunburn reaction in which the skin's response is excessive for the degree of exposure. During childhood, marked freckling develops on exposed skin along with dryness, telangiectasis and hypopigmented patches. Actinic keratoses often appear in infancy while the median age of skin cancer development is 8 years. The predominant skin malignancies are squamous and basal cell carcinomas, although the incidence of malignant melanoma is also elevated and metastatic melanoma is a cause of premature death in XP patients. Ocular abnormalities result from UV damage to the cornea and conjunctiva leading to photophobia, keratitis and scarring.

A defect in NER is diagnosed by measuring unscheduled DNA synthesis (UDS) in the patient's cultured fibroblasts. UDS occurs separately from replicative DNA synthesis and includes the generation of DNA for repair purposes. Following UV irradiation, normal cells will demonstrate an increase in UDS whereas no such response will be noted in XP fibroblasts.

In complementation studies cells from patients with different sub-types of XP can be fused to produce a 'heterokaryon' with reconstitution of a normal repair mechanism while fibroblasts from patients with the same DNA repair defect will not correct each other. The functional sub-types are called 'complementation groups'. Seven DNA excision repair-deficient complementation groups have been identified (and named XPA–XPG); each group corresponds to defects in one of the genes involved in NER. In XPA the gene responsible has been identified on chromosome 9q34. XPA protein binds specifically to damaged DNA and is critical in initiating DNA repair by the recognition of a damaged DNA adduct. XPA is the sub-type most commonly associated with severe

---

Learning points

1. Xeroderma pigmentosum (XP) should be considered in an infant presenting with an abnormally florid sunburn reaction. Erythema and blistering, which is often delayed in onset, can occur on minimal sunlight exposure.
2. The signs of accelerated photodamage and photocarcinogenesis in XP result from a genetic impairment of DNA repair.
3. In certain sub-groups of XP skin problems are associated with a degenerative neurological disorder resulting in severe functional disability.

neurological impairment as seen in our case. Although the mechanism of neuronal injury is not known, it has been proposed that transcribed genes in neuronal cells are continuously damaged by endogenous DNA-damaging agents and metabolic stress. The accumulation of unrepaired, damaged DNA impairs the synthesis of proteins necessary for neuronal survival. This results in a primary degeneration of axons leading to a loss of neurones in the cerebrum and cerebellum.

Currently, treatment of XP is centred on photoprotection in order to limit UV DNA damage and photocarcinogenesis. However, there is no effective method of slowing the associated neurological changes.

Reference

Lambert WC, Kuo H-R, Lambert MW. Xeroderma pigmentosum. *Dermatol Clin* 1995; 13: 169–203.

See also case number 25.

Case 17
A papular eruption in a patient with leukaemia

History

A 57-year-old man with chronic lymphocytic leukaemia (CLL) was referred with a rash. The patient had been diagnosed with CLL 10 years earlier and since then had received treatment with monthly courses of chlorambucil. Over the 3 months prior to referral, he had developed a widespread, pruritic skin eruption.

Clinical features

There were numerous, indurated, erythematous papules and nodules distributed widely over the face, trunk and limbs (Figure 17a). The eruption was confluent over the forehead, resulting in a large area of infiltrated erythema (Figure 17b). General examination revealed hepatosplenomegaly, axillary and inguinal lymphadenopathy.

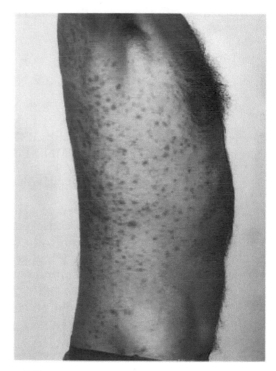

Figure 17a

Leukaemia cutis.
Multiple, monomorphic, erythematous papules are present over the torso.

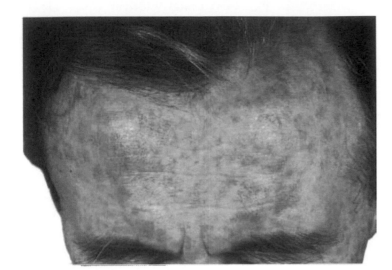

Figure 17b

Leukaemia cutis.
On the forehead there are numerous papules, which, in areas, have coalesced.

Investigations

Hb: 10.2 g/dl (11.5–15.5 g/dl), WCC: 20 × 10^9/l (4.0–11.0 × 10^9/l) [PMN: 1.3 × 10^9/l (2.0–5.0 × 10^9/l), lymphs: 17.8 × 10^9/l (1.0–3.0 × 10^9/l)], plts: 83 × 10^9/l (150–450 × 10^9/l).

Skin histopathology: Biopsy of a papule on the upper arm revealed a dense periadnexal and perivascular dermal infiltrate composed of small lymphoid cells (Figures 17c, d). Kappa (κ) and lambda (λ) immunocytochemistry demonstrated that all the cells expressed λ light chains, but were negative to κ light chains (Figure 17e).

Diagnosis

Leukaemia cutis.

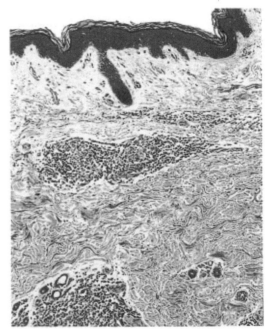

Figure 17c

Leukaemia cutis in chronic lymphocytic leukaemia.
Skin histopathology (H&E, low power). There is a dense periadnexal and perivascular infiltrate. The cells do not display epidermotropism.

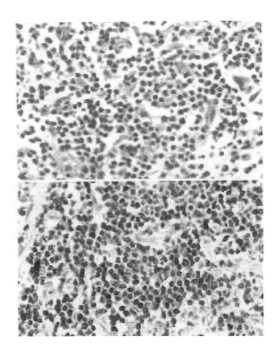

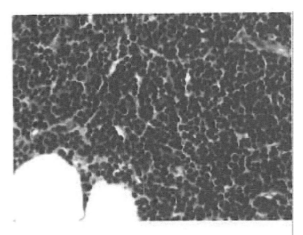

Figure 17e

Chronic lymphocytic leukaemia.
Bone marrow biopsy (high power). The bone marrow shows extensive replacement by a diffuse infiltrate of small lymphocytic cells. The features are those of CLL.

Figure 17d

Leukaemia cutis in chronic lymphocytic leukaemia.
Upper panel: Skin histopathology (H&E, high power). The infiltrate is composed of uniformly small lymphocytes.
Lower panel: Skin immunohistochemistry (high power). There is strong immunoreactivity of the lymphocytes to λ light chains, indicating monoclonality.

Treatment and progress

The patient was treated with chemotherapy consisting of cyclophosphamide, doxorubicin and vincristine. Prednisolone was omitted because of a previous episode of corticosteroid-induced hypomania. Chemotherapy resulted in a reduction in the splenomegaly and lymphadenopathy but no improvement in the rash. A 6 week course of topical nitrogen mustard had no effect on the eruption. Total skin electron-beam radiotherapy and psoralen-UVA (PUVA) photochemotherapy were declined by the patient. Finally, fludarabine was used; however, again there was no appreciable therapeutic benefit. With time, the lesions became more prominent, some developing into large violaceous nodules. The patient died from bronchopneumonia 3 years after the initial diagnosis of leukaemia cutis.

Comment

Leukaemia can be associated with various non-specific skin manifestations, such as petechiae and purpura, which are secondary to bone marrow failure. The diagnosis of leukaemia cutis (LC) is made when the eruption is secondary to infiltration of the skin with neoplastic leucocytes. The deposits are thought to result from local proliferation of leukaemic cells within the skin rather than via the migration of circulating cells from the cutaneous microvasculature.

The incidence of LC varies with the type of leukaemia, the highest prevalence being observed in myeloid leukaemias with monocytic differentiation. It occurs in 10–50% of cases of acute monocytic leukaemia, in 4–20% of cases of CLL, and in less than 10% of cases of acute lymphoblastic leukaemia and hairy cell leukaemia. The lesions take the form of red or violaceous papules, nodules or plaques. Rarely, the lesions of LC can present as bullae or figurate erythemas. In acute leukaemias and chronic lymphocytic leukaemia the lesions have a predilection for the face and extremities, while in monocytic leukaemias the entire body may be involved. LC may occur either as a late manifestation of leukaemia or, more rarely, several months before the detection of leukaemic cells in the peripheral blood, in which case it is known as aleukaemic leukaemia cutis.

The diagnosis of LC is based on the correlation of the clinical picture with haematological findings and recognition of the dominant cell type in the skin infiltrate. There is a wide spectrum of histopathological variation in LC depending on the type of leukaemia and degree of differentiation. In CLL there is an infiltrate of small lymphocytes involving the dermis and sometimes the subcutis. There is often perivascular and periadnexal aggregation, and adnexal destruction may be a feature. In chronic myelomonocytic leukaemia (CMML) the cell population is more pleomorphic, with granulocytes in varying stages of differentiation. In CLL, where normal and neoplastic lymphocytes are morphologically identical, immunocytochemical staining with κ and λ surface markers is useful to determine

> # Learning points
>
> 1. The development of multiple, infiltrated, erythematous papules or nodules in a patient with leukaemia is suggestive of leukaemia cutis (LC). The diagnosis should be confirmed by appropriate analysis of a skin biopsy.
> 2. LC usually occurs as a late manifestation of leukaemia. However, rarely, it can present several months before the detection of leukaemic cells in the peripheral blood, in which case it is known as aleukaemic LC.
> 3. In a patient with leukaemia it is important to distinguish LC from other cutaneous lesions since LC is associated with a poor prognosis.

monoclonality. As well as light-chain restriction, positive staining to CD5 and CD23 is consistently found in CLL.

LC is associated with a poor prognosis and therapy should be directed to the underlying leukaemia. However, therapy sufficient to induce bone marrow remission only may not control the LC. The skin may also act as a sanctuary site for leukaemic cells so that the bone marrow may be re-seeded following chemotherapy. Therefore a combination of chemotherapy and total skin electron beam radiotherapy is now recommended.

Reference

Ratnam KV, Khor CLJ, Su WPD. Leukaemia cutis. *Dermatol Clin* 1994; 12: 419–31.

See also case number 32.

Case 18
A polycyclic rash in a patient with epilepsy

History

A 25-year-old woman, who was an in-patient under the care of the neuro-psychiatrists, was referred with a widespread eruption. She had longstanding epilepsy secondary to a benign neuro-developmental lesion, which was exacerbated by chronic excessive intake of alcohol. Over the previous few months her epilepsy had worsened and her anticonvulsant therapy (carbamazepine, lamotrigine) had been increased. Some days after the change in her medication she developed an acute dermatosis.

Clinical findings

Examination revealed an erythematous, inflammatory eruption predominantly affecting the back, chest, neck and proximal limbs. The lesions were circinate and annular, some coalescing to give a polycyclic configuration (Figure 18a). There was some surface scaling on many of the lesions, whilst a few were eroded (Figure 18b). On the face there was telangiectatic erythema (Figure 18c). There was livedo reticularis on the arms and legs. The eruption spared the axillae and groins. There was no mucous membrane involvement. General examination was normal.

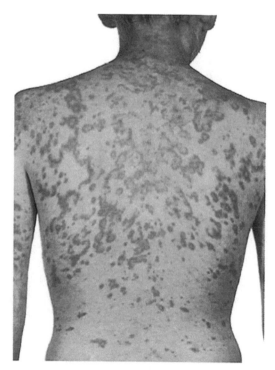

Figure 18a

Sub-acute cutaneous lupus erythematosus. There is an eruption on the upper trunk and proximal arms characterized by annular, circinate and polycyclic lesions.

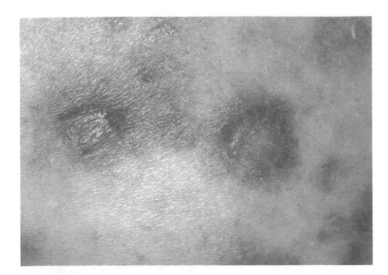

Figure 18b

Sub-acute cutaneous lupus erythematosus.
Active lesions in SCLE may become eroded.

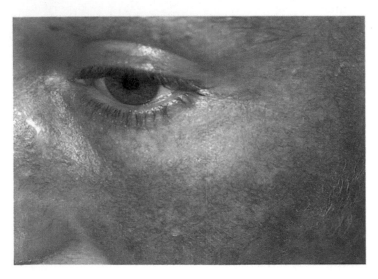

Figure 18c

Sub-acute cutaneous lupus erythematosus.
Telangiectatic erythema of the face often occurs in SCLE.

Investigations

FBC: normal, U&E: normal, ESR: 26 mm/hr (1–10 mm/hr).

GGT: 210 IU/l (5–55 IU/l), AST: 104 IU/l (10–50 IU/l), ALP: 63 IU/l (30–120 IU/l), bilirubin: 14 µmol/l (3–20 µmol/l).

ANA: negative.

ENA: Ro positive; La, Sm, RNP, Jo-1, Scl-70 all negative.

Anti-histone antibodies: negative.

Complement: normal.

Skin histopathology: Biopsy of a lesion on the back demonstrated a lymphocytic infiltrate in the superficial dermis with basal vacuolation and degeneration of keratinocytes. Satellite cell necrosis was also seen (Figure 18d). Direct immunofluorescence revealed a linear deposition of IgM at the dermo–epidermal junction (Figure 18e).

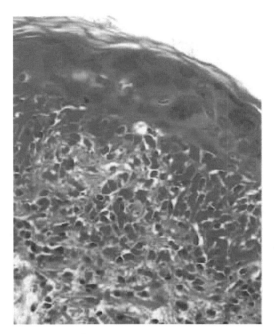

Figure 18d

Sub-acute cutaneous lupus erythematosus.
Skin histopathology (H&E, high power).
There is an interface dermatitis with
numerous intraepithelial necrotic
keratinocytes, basal vacuolation and a
dense dermal lymphocytic infiltrate.

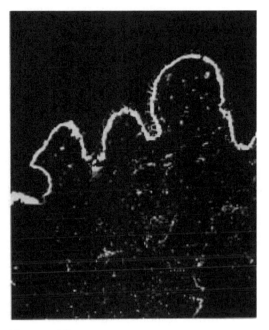

Figure 18e

Sub-acute cutaneous lupus erythematosus.
Skin direct immunofluorescence. There is a
linear deposition of IgM at the dermo–epidermal
junction, a pattern consistent with lupus
erythematosus.

Diagnosis

Sub-acute cutaneous lupus erythematosus.

Treatment and progress

Substitution of carbamazepine by clonaze-
pam caused no improvement in the rash and
resulted in poor control of her epilepsy.

Initially, she improved with prednisolone 30
mg daily along with the use of a superpotent
topical corticosteroid and a high-protection-
factor topical sunscreen. However, following
discharge and with reduction in the dose of
prednisolone, the eruption relapsed and she
was commenced on hydroxychloroquine

200 mg twice daily, mepacrine 100 mg on
alternate days and intramuscular methylprednisolone 120 mg every 4 weeks. Long-term
control of the dermatosis proved difficult.

Comment

Sub-acute cutaneous lupus erythematosus
(SCLE) is a distinct dermatosis within the
spectrum of LE skin disease. SCLE usually
presents as a papulosquamous dermatosis
showing an annular or polycyclic configuration, often in individuals with skin type I or
II. The typical figurate eruption has a
predilection for sun-exposed sites, particularly the upper body and proximal arms,
while the development of a photodistributed

erythema occurs in approximately 50% of cases. A high co-incidence of polymorphic light eruption may confuse the true incidence of photosensitivity. Other associations include discoid lupus erythematosus, livedo reticularis, non-scarring alopecia, Raynaud's phenomenon and mucous membrane ulcers.

Anti-Ro antibodies are found in approximately 70% of patients with SCLE and anti-La in around 40%. The role of these antibodies has not yet been fully elucidated; however, ultraviolet light causes increased Ro and La expression on keratinocytes, which may then offer a target for activated lymphocytes. However, this hypothesis does not explain the presence of SCLE lesions on chronically covered skin.

The major histocompatability complex (MHC) on chromosome 6 plays an important role in immune responses, and certain MHC class II loci are thought to be particularly associated with SCLE. These include HLA-A1, B8, DR3, DQ1, DQ2, DRw52 and C4null. These loci control not only the presence or absence of an anti-Ro response but also the level of response. DR3 is thought to be associated particularly with the annular lesions of SCLE. DR2 similarly has been associated with a later onset and with the papulosquamous variety of SCLE. Inherited deficiencies of C2 and C4 have also been strongly linked with SCLE.

Certain drugs, including antihypertensives (e.g. hydrochlorothiazide, calcium channel blockers and ACE inhibitors) and anti-fungals (griseofulvin and terbinafine), have been reported as important triggers for SCLE. An iatrogenic cause must therefore be considered in a patient presenting with typical clinical features of SCLE who has been recently exposed to an implicated drug. Positive serology to Ro or La is commonly, but not always, found in these cases. Although our patient had been taking carbamazepine and lamotrigine for a number of years, the dose of both drugs had been increased just prior to her presentation. Anti-

> **Learning points**
>
> 1. The appearance of an annular and polycyclic eruption on the upper trunk in the context of abnormal photosensitivity is suggestive of sub-acute cutaneous lupus erythematosus (SCLE). The majority of cases have an associated positive extractable nuclear antigen (ENA), with antibodies to Ro or La.
> 2. SCLE can be triggered by drugs, the most commonly implicated being: anti-hypertensives (thiazides, calcium channel blockers, ACE inhibitors) and anti-fungals (griseofulvin, terbinafine).
> 3. Skin biopsy of lesional skin will demonstrate the typical features of cutaneous LE while direct immunofluorescence will display immunoglobulin deposited at the dermo–epidermal junction.

convulsants have not been associated with drug-induced SCLE; however, the temporal relationship in our case suggests a causal link in the provocation of her eruption.

The eruption of SCLE can often be controlled with topical or systemic corticosteroids. Second-line agents with steroid-sparing activity include anti-malarials, cyclosporin, oral gold and thalidomide. In a small number of reported patients with resistant disease treatment with intravenous immunoglobulin has been successful. Sun avoidance and the use of a high-protection-factor sunscreen is important in those with a photosensitive component.

Reference

Callen JP, Klein J. Subacute cutaneous lupus erythematosus: clinical, serologic, immunogenetic and therapeutic considerations. *Arthritis Rheum* 1988; 31: 1007–13.

See also case number 2.

Case 19
Flexural papules, thirst and polyuria

History

A 34-year-old man, originally from India, first presented with a 6-month history of excessive thirst and polyuria. Over this period he had also noticed loss of libido and the appearance of skin lesions in his armpits. His symptoms were investigated but results were inconclusive and no definitive diagnosis was made. A year later he was admitted acutely with malaise, vomiting and severe thirst. Biochemical investigation showed hyperosmolar, non-ketotic diabetes mellitus, which was treated with insulin and fluid replacement. In spite of correction of the hyperglycaemia, the patient's thirst and polyuria persisted. In addition, it was noted that the cutaneous eruption had extended. A dermatology opinion was requested.

Clinical findings

Inspection of the skin revealed a symmetrical eruption of multiple, monomorphic yellow-brown papules in the axillae, groins, antecubital fossae, neck and eyelids (Figures 19a–b). Tan-coloured papules were also present on the buccal mucosa. Axillary and pubic hair was diminished.

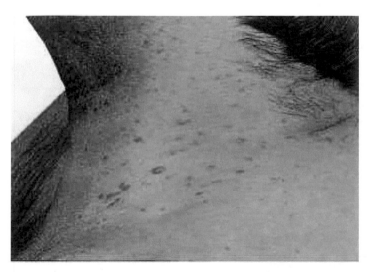

Figure 19a

Xanthoma disseminatum.
Multiple yellow-brown papules, resembling xanthomata were present on the neck.

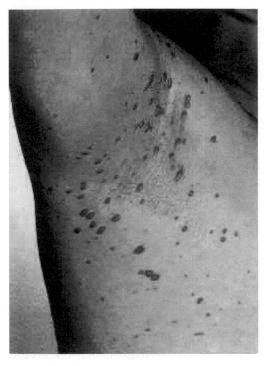

Figure 19b

Xanthoma disseminatum.
Lesions were also found in the axilla.
Axillary hair was markedly diminished.

Investigations

Skin histopathology: Biopsy of an axillary lesion demonstrated a dermal infiltrate consisting of histiocytes, foam cells and giant cells. Multinucleated giant cells, in particular Touton giant cells, were scattered in the upper dermis (Figure 19c).

Pituitary stimulation tests confirmed panhypopituitarism and diabetes insipidus.

Diagnosis

Xanthoma disseminatum.

Treatment and progress

One year after the patient was diagnosed with xanthoma disseminatum he suffered a myocardial infarction and died. The postmortem findings confirmed almost total

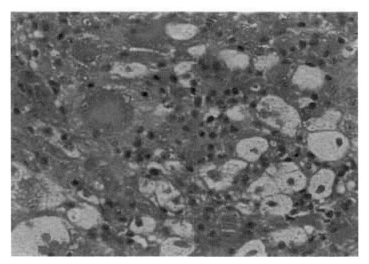

Figure 19c

Xanthoma disseminatum.
Skin histopathology (H&E, high power). There is a mixed dermal infiltrate of histiocytes, foamy macrophages, lymphocytes and a number of Touton multinucleated giant cells

occlusion of the proximal left anterior descending and circumflex coronary arteries. In the trachea there were small sub-epithelial infiltrates of histiocytes, lymphocytes and giant cells. The pituitary stalk was widened and contained a histiocytic-rich infiltrate. The posterior lobe of the pituitary showed extensive fibrosis with an infiltrate of histiocytes, some showing the beginnings of giant cell formation.

Comment

Xanthoma disseminatum (XD) is a rare, non-Langerhans, class II histiocytosis that appears to be sporadic and occurs predominantly in young adult males. The cutaneous manifestations are usually prominent early in the disease, but diabetes insipidus due to involvement of the pituitary stalk occurs in 40% of cases and may be the presenting feature. Further central nervous system involvement may cause epilepsy, hydocephalus or ataxia.

Typically, the eruption commences with enlarging yellow-brown papules on the trunk or face, which develop into xanthomatous plaques involving the flexures, with particular predilection for the axillae. Buccal mucous membrane involvement occurs in up to 50% of cases whilst lesions may also affect the mucous membranes of the oropharynx, respiratory tract and conjunctivae.

Histologically, XD is characterized by infiltration of the dermis with foamy histiocytes, giant cells and leucocytes. The histiocytes in XD have irregular scalloped borders with extensive cytoplasm and ovoid vesicular nuclei. In older lesions Touton giant cells may be observed. At the ultrastructural level histiocytes contain membrane-bound fat droplets. Lipid deposition in lesional tissue is a secondary event in XD. However, cases have been described, like ours, in which concomitant hyperlipidaemia and atherosclerosis is prominent and may be associated with fatal cardiovascular sequelae.

Most commonly, XD follows a benign course with lesions continuing to develop for up to 40 years. Occasionally the condition is progressive with multi-system involvement. Treatment for XD is unsatisfactory, although some degree of spontaneous resolution can occur with lesions clearing to leave atrophic scars.

Learning points

1. The development of xanthomatous papules occurring in association with diabetes insipidus is highly suggestive of xanthoma disseminatum (XD).
2. The diagnosis of XD can be made on the skin biopsy, which demonstrates a dermal infiltrate consisting of histiocytes, foam cells and multi-nucleated giant cells, in particular Touton giant cells.
3. XD usually follows a benign course. However, some cases can result in death from involvement of the respiratory tract or central nervous system.

Reference

Zelger B, Burgdorf WH. The cutaneous 'histiocytoses'. *Adv Dermatol* 2001; 17: 77–114.

See also case numbers 6, 35, 44.

Case 20
Facial plaques and fever

History

A 66-year-old woman presented with a 10-day history of a facial dematosis. The eruption commenced as a number of discrete papules, which rapidly expanded and coalesced to form three large, painful plaques. The eruption was associated with a fever. There was no relevant past medical history.

Clinical features

The patient was febrile (38.6°C). Examination of the skin revealed erythematous plaques on the forehead, right cheek and left cheek, each measuring 4–8 cm in diameter (Figure 20a). The lesions had a firm, deep-red margin and a pseudovesicular surface with some crusting (Figure 20b). There was no regional lymphadenopathy. The remainder of the general examination was unremarkable.

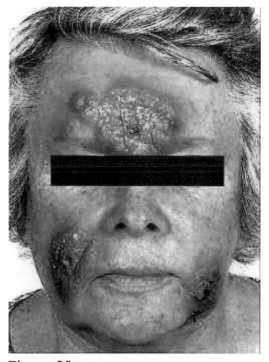

Figure 20a

Sweet's syndrome.
There are large inflamed plaques on the forehead and both cheeks.

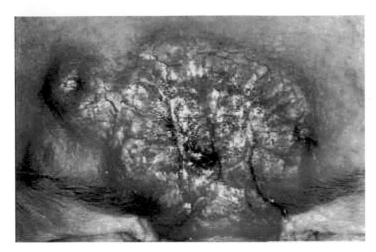

Figure 20b

Sweet's syndrome.
A close-up of the forehead lesion demonstrates a deep-red plaque with surface crusting and pseudovesiculation.

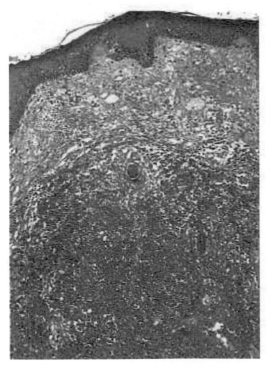

Figure 20c

Sweet's syndrome.
Skin histopathology (H&E, low power).
There is a dense infiltrate of inflammatory cells within the mid and lower dermis.
The upper dermis is oedematous while the overlying epidermis is normal.

Investigations

Hb: 13.9 g/dl (11.5–15.5 g/dl), WCC: 15.6 × 10^9/l (4.0–11.0), PMN: 12.5 × 10^9/l (2.0–7.5 × 10^9/l), plts: 454 × 10^9/l (150–450 × 10^9/l). ESR: 44 mm/hr (1–10 mm/hr).

U&E: normal, LFT: normal, immunoglobulins: normal, serum protein electrophoresis: normal.

Autoantibodies: negative, RF: negative.

Skin histopathology: Biopsy of a cheek lesion showed oedema of the papillary dermis with a dense infiltrate in the mid-dermis composed predominantly of neutrophils with occasional lymphocytes and eosinophils (Figures 20c, d).

Diagnosis

Sweet's syndrome (acute febrile neutrophilic dermatosis).

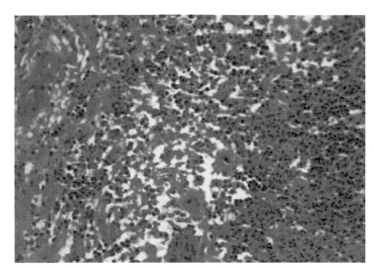

Figure 20d

Sweet's syndrome.
Skin histopathology (H&E, high power). The dermal inflammatory cell infiltrate is composed predominantly of neutrophils.

Treatment and progress

A bone marrow biopsy, performed to exclude an underlying haematological malignancy, was normal. The patient was commenced on prednisolone 30 mg once daily. There was a good response to high-dose corticosteroid with complete resolution of the lesions. However, the eruption recurred as the dose of prednisolone was lowered below 15 mg. Dapsone 50 mg once daily was added, which permitted further gradual reduction in the prednisolone. Two years after presentation both drugs were discontinued and over 5 subsequent years of follow-up there was no relapse in the patient's dermatosis.

Comment

In Robert Sweet's original 1964 description of acute febrile neutrophilic dermatosis eight women presented with a skin disease characterized by recurrent painful inflammatory plaques associated with fever, peripheral neutrophilia and, histopathologically, a neutrophil-rich dermal infiltrate. In each case the disorder responded promptly to treatment with systemic glucocorticoids. The literature on Sweet's syndrome has identified a strong association with haematological malignancy (commonly acute myeloid leukaemia), however, 80% of cases appear to occur in isolation. The aetiology of the idiopathic cases remains unclear; however, a number of patients report a preceding febrile upper respiratory tract infection, which suggests that the ensuing dermatosis may represent a hypersensitivity reaction to bacterial or viral antigen. Recombinant granulocyte–macrophage colony-stimulating factor (GM-CSF), a drug used to reduce the duration of neutropenia in chemotherapy-induced marrow failure, can induce an eruption clinically and histopathologically identical to Sweet's syndrome. This association identifies a potential role for endogenous neutrophil-specific leukotactic factors in the pathogenesis of all forms of Sweet's syndrome.

Clinically, the initial skin lesions of Sweet's syndrome are dark red papules or nodules, occurring most commonly on the face, neck and arms, which tend to coalesce forming well-demarcated inflammatory plaques. Established lesions are tender and often painful, and may demonstrate a pseudovesicular surface secondary to dermal oedema. Systemic symptoms usually accompany the skin eruption, most usually, fever, arthralgia and malaise. However, not all cases of Sweet's syndrome express the whole spectrum of clinical features, and both fever and neutrophilia may be absent.

As well as responding to glucocorticoids, other agents used successfully either singly or in combination with glucocorticoids are colchicine, dapsone, clofazimine and potassium iodide. A number of patients may be difficult to wean off therapy and clinical relapse in Sweet's syndrome is not uncommon.

Learning points

1. Sweet's syndrome presents as an acute eruption of multiple, deep-red nodules or plaques accompanied by fever, arthralgia and malaise.
2. Histologically, the lesions are characterized by a dense dermal infiltrate of neutrophils, while blood tests demonstrate a circulating neutrophilia.
3. Approximately 20% of cases are associated with haematological malignancy, commonly acute myeloid leukaemia.

Reference

Callen JP. Neutrophilic dermatoses. *Dermatol Clin* 2002; 20: 409–19.

See also case number 13.

Case 21
Generalized thickening of the skin following bone marrow transplantation

History

A 30-year-old woman was diagnosed with acute myeloid leukaemia and underwent a matched unrelated allogeneic bone marrow transplant. A year later, following a relapse, she received donor lymphocyte infusions. Within 12 months she began to develop an illness consisting of rash, diarrhoea and weight loss. Initial skin lesions consisted of erythematous patches with hypopigmented atrophic centres (Figure 21a). Over the next 2 years the areas of involvement expanded with generalized thickening and stiffening of her skin. In addition, she developed dry eyes and a dry mouth.

Clinical findings

The patient was thin. Examination of the skin revealed extensive sclerodermatous areas on the trunk and limbs, which displayed mottled hyperpigmentation (Figure 21b). The skin of the digits was waxy and tight. On the lower abdomen there were large pits secondary to loss of subcutaneous fat. Flexion deformities were present at the elbows, wrists, knees and ankles (Figure 21c). She had a sicca syndrome involving eyes and mouth.

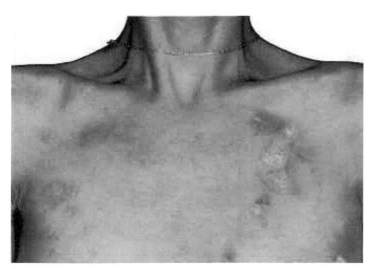

Figure 21a

Early sclerodermoid GVHD.
Three months after presentation there were a few sclerotic plaques on the upper chest, each surrounded by a faint erythematous margin. The remainder of the skin was normal.

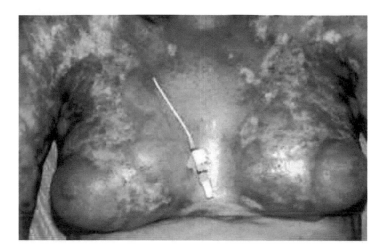

Figure 21b

Late sclerodermoid GVHD.
Two years after presentation there
were widespread areas of sclerosis
characterized by hyperpigmented and
hypopigmented, indurated skin. A
Hickman line has been inserted for
venous access.

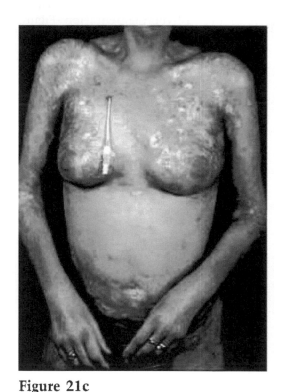

Figure 21c

Sclerodermoid GVHD.
Sclerodermoid changes are present over
the chest, abdomen and proximal limbs.
There are contractures causing fixed
flexion of the elbows, wrists and fingers.

Investigations

Skin histopathology: Biopsy of the chest skin
showed epidermal atrophy and a grossly
thickened, sclerotic dermis composed of
expanded bundles of pale hyalinized collagen. Dermal sclerosis had replaced adnexal
structures, including hair follicles and sweat
glands (Figure 21d).

Diagnosis

**Chronic   sclerodermoid   graft-versus-host-
disease.**

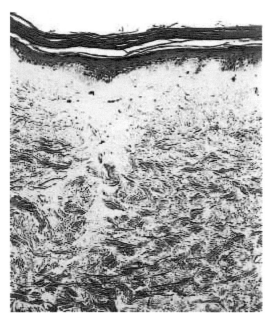

Figure 21d

Sclerodermoid GVHD.
Skin histopathology (H&E, low power).
There is epidermal atrophy with pigment incontinence. Throughout the full thickness of the dermis there is sclerosis with expanded bundles of pale hyalinized collagen. Adnexal structures, such as hair follicles and sweat glands, have been lost.

Treatment and progress

Severe sclerodermatous skin changes resulted in restricted function of arms, hands and legs. Intestinal involvement by graft-versus-host disease (GVHD) caused malabsorption while lung involvement led to bronchiolitis obliterans. In an attempt to treat the GVHD, the patient has received the following therapies: cyclosporin, tacrolimus, prednisolone, mycophenolate mofetil, thalidomide, intravenous immunoglobulin, anti-interleukin-2 receptor antibody and extracorporeal photopheresis. None of these have significantly modified the course of her illness. The leukaemia has remained in remission.

Comment

In graft-versus-host disease (GVHD) the introduction of immunologically active foreign cells (graft) induces epithelial damage in the recipient (host). The disorder is mediated by donor T lymphocytes that are activated by exposure to histocompatibility antigens on recipient tissues. GVHD occurs most commonly following the transplantation of haematopoietic stem cells and it develops in 30–60% of patients receiving allogeneic transplants for the treatment of haematological malignancies. However, leukaemia relapse rates are considerably lower in patients who develop GVHD, suggesting that donor immune cells may eradicate residual malignant haematopoietic cells (the graft-versus-leukaemia effect). The incidence of GVHD increases with the use of unmatched transplants and in those who receive donor lymphocyte infusions, as in our patient.

GVHD occurs in an acute and a chronic form, each with distinctive clinical features. Cutaneous signs are invariably present and often the first sign of the disease. Acute GVHD usually occurs within 1–8 weeks after transplantation and is a pathological process that specifically targets epithelia of the skin, gastrointestinal tract and intrahepatic bile ducts. Chronic GVHD usually arises within 3–16 months post transplantation. Chronic disease occurs either as an extension of acute GVHD, or following a period of quiescence, or arises de novo. The clinical manifestations of chronic GVHD are similar to those of the autoimmune collagen vascular diseases. The cutaneous eruption typically begins with the development of pruritic violaceous papules which may enlarge or coalesce to form scaly erythematous plaques, so-called 'chronic lichenoid GVHD'. Chronic GVHD can also take a sclerodermoid form, as in our case, in which hyper- or hypopigmented plaques resembling morphoea arise, usually on the trunk and proximal limbs. These lesions may enlarge to form widespread areas of brawny induration. In sclerodermoid GVHD the disease can extend to the subcutaneous tissue and fascia to produce disabling joint contractures that are a major cause of morbidity. Involvement of the salivary lacrimal glands can cause a sicca syndrome while lichen planus-like reticulate plaques can occur on the buccal mucosae. Chronic GVHD of the liver causes portal tract fibrosis that leads to cirrhosis. Less often, a bronchiolitis obliterans develops, a condition that carries a grave prognosis.

Treatment of chronic GVHD is unsatisfactory, with little reported improvement despite the use of a variety of aggressive immunosuppressive therapies.

Learning points

1. 30–60% of patients receiving an allogeneic haematopoietic stem cell transplant for haematological malignancy will develop graft-versus-host disease (GVHD), a multi-system disorder of skin, gut and liver.
2. The incidence and severity of GVHD is increased by the use of donor lymphocyte infusions.
3. Chronic sclerodermoid GVHD can cause profound disability through widespread cutaneous sclerosis and associated joint contractures.

Reference

Lee SJ, Vogelsang G, Flowers ME. Chronic graft-versus-host disease. *Biol Blood Marrow Transplant* 2003; 4: 215–33.

See also case numbers 7, 26.

Case 22
Pruritic plaques in pregnancy

History

A 23-year-old primigravida presented at 28 weeks' gestation with a 6-day history of a widespread, pruritic eruption. The lesions developed initially on periumbilical skin and subsequently spread to involve the trunk and proximal limbs. She had a past history of Graves' disease and alopecia universalis, the latter having responded successfully to a course of psoralen-UVA (PUVA) administered 3 years previously. She gave a strong family history of autoimmune disorders, her mother suffering from primary biliary cirrhosis, hypothyroidism and alopecia areata, whilst two of her siblings were also known to have autoimmune thyroid disease.

Clinical findings

There were numerous erythematous, urticated plaques on the abdomen, chest and proximal limbs (Figure 22a). Some lesions had a target-like morphology. A few of the lesions on her legs had blistered (Figure 22b). Mucous membrane examination was normal.

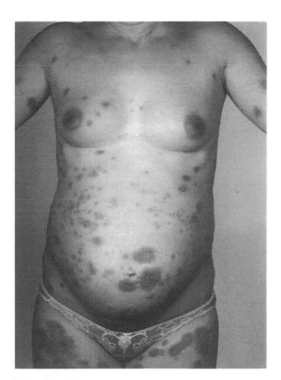

Figure 22a

Pemphigoid gestationis.
There are widespread urticated plaques on the abdomen, particularly involving periumbilical skin.

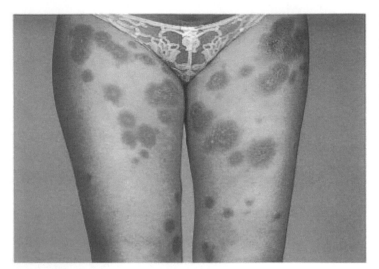

Figure 22b

Pemphigoid gestationis.
The lesions on the thighs
demonstrate a targetoid morphology,
with some showing incipient
blistering.

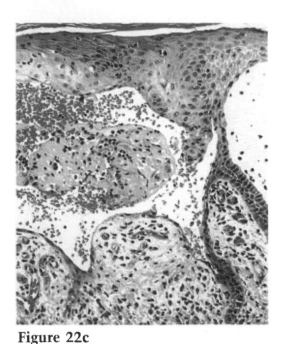

Figure 22c

Pemphigoid gestationis.
Skin histopathology (H&E, high power).
There is a sub-epidermal blister with
eosinophils in the dermis and blister
cavity. There is early epidermal
regeneration at the blister base.

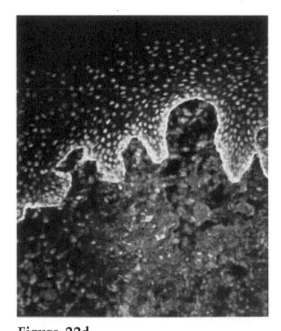

Figure 22d

Pemphigoid gestationis.
Direct immunofluorescence of perilesional
skin showing bright linear C3 deposition
at the basement membrane zone.

Investigations

Skin histopathology: Biopsy through a blister demonstrated a sub-epidermal split with eosinophils in the blister fluid and an oedematous upper dermis containing a mixed perivascular infiltrate including eosinophils (Figure 22c).

Direct immunofluorescence of perilesional skin demonstrated linear C3 deposition along the basement membrane zone (Figure 22d).

Indirect immunofluorescence demonstrated positive C3 immunoreactivity at the basement membrane zone.

Diagnosis

Pemphigoid gestationis.

Treatment and progress

The patient was commenced on prednisolone 40 mg once daily, with rapid resolution of the skin lesions. Over the remaining weeks of her pregnancy the prednisolone was gradually reduced and was discontinued by week 38 of pregnancy. She delivered a healthy baby at 40 weeks; however, there was a slight flare of the patient's eruption in the first post-partum week. This was successfully managed with a superpotent topical corticosteroid. Three years later, during the second trimester of her second pregnancy, the patient again developed pruritic, urticated plaques on the abdominal skin. Biopsy confirmed pemphigoid gestationis and the eruption was fully controlled with topical corticosteroid alone.

Comment

Pemphigoid gestationis (PG) is a rare autoimmune bullous disease, which is estimated to complicate 1 in 40 000–60 000 pregnancies. PG may develop at any time from 9 weeks' gestation to 1 week post-partum but usually presents during the second and third trimesters. The disease is likely to recur in subsequent pregnancies, often with an earlier onset and more florid expression.

PG typically presents with pruritic erythematous urticated papules and plaques, which may become annular or target-like. Progression to blisters on erythematous skin usually follows a pre-bullous phase. In 90% of patients the eruption commences on periumbilical skin, with later spread to the chest, abdomen, arms, legs, palms and soles. Occasionally, there is spontaneous remission of the disease during the latter part of pregnancy, only to flare at the time of delivery. Up to 10% of infants born to mothers with PG have cutaneous lesions. Transient urticarial or vesicular lesions are most common and resolve within 3 weeks as transferred maternal antibodies are catabolized.

Differentiation of PG from other pregnancy dermatoses is usually not difficult once blisters have developed. However, in its initial phase the eruption may be confused with polymorphic eruption of pregnancy (previously known as pruritic, urticated papules and plaques of pregnancy, PUPPP). In contrast to PG, polymorphic eruption of pregnancy typically develops during the third trimester in primiparous women and is characterized by prominent involvement of abdominal striae. Other diseases that should be considered in the differential diagnosis include other autoimmune bullous dermatoses and erythema multiforme.

There is a recognized association of PG with other autoimmune disorders. A study of

87 patients with PG reported a 14% incidence of Graves' disease. Interestingly, both PG and Graves' disease are known to be associated with the HLA-DR3 antigen, which suggests a shared immunopathogenetic pathway. Our patient had a past history of both Graves' disease and alopecia areata and a strong family history of autoimmune disease. A hereditary susceptibility to autoimmune disorders is recognized, with a 25% incidence of autoimmune diseases in the relatives of patients with PG.

The diagnostic immunohistochemical finding in PG is linear deposition of C3, with or without IgG, along the basement membrane zone of perilesional skin. A circulating PG factor is detected in approximately 25% of patients using an indirect immunofluorescence technique. With the use of sodium chloride split skin, the PG factor will demonstrate epidermal (rather than dermal) binding. Immunoprecipitation studies have demonstrated that the majority of PG sera recognize the 180 kDa bullous pemphigoid antigen 2 (BPAg2), while some also react to the 230 kDa BPAg1.

In mild cases of PG the use of superpotent topical corticosteroids combined with systemic antihistamines and emollients is often adequate. However, once bullae have developed it is necessary to use systemic corticosteroids, such as prednisolone, with disease control usually being achieved at a dose of 40 mg once daily. Thereafter, the dosage should be gradually reduced to the minimum effective dose. As post-partum exacerbations are frequent it is often recommended that the steroid dose is increased temporarily immediately after delivery.

> ## Learning points
>
> 1. Pemphigoid gestationis (PG) is an uncommon disorder of pregnancy. The eruption is very pruritic and initially urticarial before becoming bullous.
> 2. It commences around the umbilicus and spreads across the abdomen and on to the limbs. It reappears with each subsequent pregnancy, often with an earlier onset.
> 3. Direct immunofluorescence showing deposits of C3 at the basement membrane is diagnostic, while a circulating PG factor (basement membrane autoantibody) is detected in approximately 25% of patients.

Reference

Jenkins RE, Hern S, Black MM. Clinical features and management of 87 patients with pemphigoid gestationis. *Clin Exp Derm* 1999; 24: 255–9.

See also case number 9.

Case 23
Multiple painless ulcers in a traveller

History

A 25-year-old man presented with a 3-week history of multiple sores developing on his face, legs and feet. The lesions were painless but were gradually increasing in size. Five weeks earlier he had returned from a prolonged trip to Brazil, where he had been working as a map-maker in the Amazon forest.

Clinical features

There were six lesions in total: one on the forehead, four on the legs and one on the left foot. The facial lesion was an eroded plaque with overlying crust, the lesions on the lower limbs were well-circumscribed, deep ulcers with erythematous margins, each measuring 1–3 cm in diameter (Figure 23a). There was also a painful, boil-like nodule on the left calf (Figure 23b).

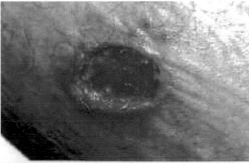
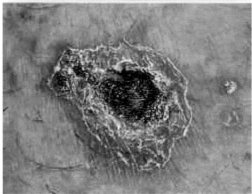

Figure 23a

South American leishmaniasis.
Upper panel: There is a well-circumscribed deep ulcer on the skin of the right calf.
Lower: There is an ulcer with overlying crust on the left thigh.

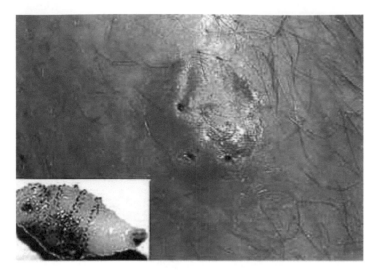

Figure 23b

Myiasis.
A boil-like nodule on the left calf with three punctate orifices.
Inset: the botfly larva (*Dermatobia hominis*) which emerged after the puncta were occluded. Encircling the bulbous end of the larva are rows of spines that keep the maggot lodged within the skin.

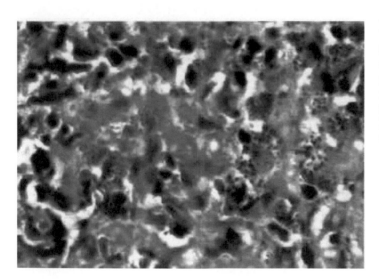

Figure 23c

South American leishmaniasis.
Skin histopathology (Giemsa, high power). There is a mixed infiltrate of macrophages and lymphocytes. Large numbers of amastigotes (Leishman–Donovan bodies) are present within the cytoplasm of the macrophages.

Investigations

Skin histopathology: Biopsy of an ulcer demonstrated keratotic debris overlying the dermis that contained a dense inflammatory cell infiltrate composed predominantly of macrophages, as well as lymphocytes, plasma cells and occasional giant cells. Within the macrophages were numerous intracytoplasmic amastigotes (Leishman–Donovan bodies) (Figure 23c).

Diagnosis

South American leishmaniasis and myiasis.

Treatment and progress

The patient was treated with a 10-day course of intravenous sodium stibogluconate

800 mg per day. This resulted in clearance of all the lesions except for the painful nodule on the calf of the left leg. This lesion, which was noted to be pulsating, had three punctate orifices. Myiasis was diagnosed and the puncta occluded with vaseline. Some hours later a larva emerged from the nodule.

Comment

The leishmaniases are a collection of chronic diseases caused by several species of the genus *Leishmania*, a haemoflagellate protozoan. Cutaneous leishmaniasis is endemic in the forested country of Central and South America and is caused by protozoa from the *L. braziliensis* and *L. mexicana* complexes, transmitted by the bite of an infected sandfly of the *Lutzomyia* spp. Man is only an 'accidental' host and is usually the end of the transmission chain, playing no important part in the maintenance of the *Leishmania* life cycle. Small forest rodents are the principle natural hosts for most species of New World *Leishmania*. In the non-immune subject there is an incubation period of between two weeks and several months from the time of being bitten by an infected sandfly until the development of a small inflammatory papule at the site of the bite. Thereafter, the lesion tends to develop into an ulcer, which is typically painless. Regional lymphadenopathy may occur but is seldom marked. Clinical forms of leishmaniasis encountered in South America include localized cutaneous disease, diffuse cutaneous disease and mucocutaneous leishmaniasis. Our patient with ulcers on a variety of anatomical sites (diffuse disease) corresponds to numerous inoculation bites.

Leishmania braziliensis is found in the humid jungle regions of northern South America, where our patient was working. The prompt diagnosis and adequate treatment of *L. braziliensis* cases is important because up to 40% of patients infected with this strain progress to nasopharyngeal mucocutaneous involvement: 50% of mucosal lesions develop within 2 years of the appearance of the skin lesion, and 90% within 10 years. The aggressive nature of this from of leishmaniasis may ultimately result in destruction of the nose, palate and lips.

There is no prophylaxis against infection other than the use of insect repellants and protective clothing. Travellers to areas where *L. braziliensis* is endemic should be aware of the importance of obtaining adequate treatment if lesions occur.

Myiasis is the infestation of body tissues by the larvae of Diptera (two-winged flies). *Dermatobia hominis* (human botfly) is found in areas of high temperature and humidity and is the commonest cause of furuncular myiasis in South America. The female botfly deposits her eggs on the abdomen of an insect vector, such as a mosquito; the eggs are introduced into the host when the vector

---

Learning points

1. Leishmaniasis should be suspected in a traveller recently returned from an endemic area in South America who presents with atypical skin ulcers. The diagnosis is made by finding amastigotes in a biopsy of lesional skin.
2. If left untreated, infection with *L. braziliensis* can progress to mucocutaneous nasopharyngeal leishmaniasis.
3. Patients can harbour more than one tropical infection. Human botfly myiasis should be considered as a cause of a boil-like lesion in a patient who has recently returned from visiting the tropical forested areas of South America.

takes a blood meal. If undisturbed, larval development lasts approximately 50–60 days, following which the larva emerges, drops to the ground and pupates. Clinically, cutaneous myiasis develops as a painful, boil-like lesion with a central punctum on the exposed skin of the face, arms and legs. The posterior end of the larva, equipped with spiracles for breathing, is sometimes visible in the punctum. Once the larva has emerged the lesion resolves. Methods of treatment include occluding the punctum with vaseline or some other grease, which provokes the larva to migrate out. Surgical extraction is also curative.

Reference

Bouree P, Belec L. Leishmaniasis: report of 33 cases and a review of the literature. *Comp Immunol Microbiol Infect Dis* 1993; 16: 251–65.

See also case number 45.

Case 24
A pigmented plaque on the knee

History

A 28-year-old man presented with a rapidly enlarging lesion on the right knee. Eight months earlier the patient had received a combined kidney-and-pancreas transplant for end-stage renal failure secondary to diabetic nephropathy. His post-transplant immuno-suppressive medication consisted of prednisolone, tacrolimus and azathioprine. Prior to the development of the skin lesion, he remembered sustaining a splinter injury to the right knee when kneeling on an exposed floorboard.

Clinical findings

On examination of the right knee, there was a 3 cm diameter plaque, which was pigmented peripherally (Figure 24a). The lesion was firm on palpation and non-tender. There was a tiny satellite lesion adjacent to the main plaque. There was no regional lymphadenopathy.

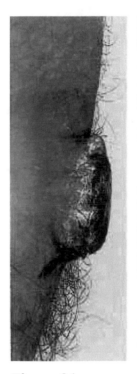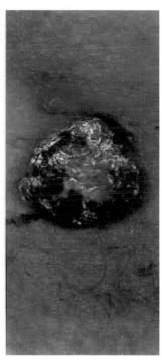

Figure 24a

Phaeohyphomycosis.
There is a plaque on the skin of the right knee with a pigmented periphery. This developed at the site of minor trauma from a wood splinter in a transplant recipient receiving tacrolimus and azathioprine.

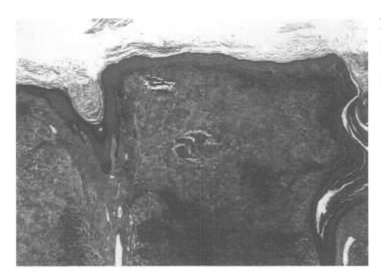

Figure 24b

Phaeohyphomycosis.
Skin histopathology (H&E, low power). There is a chronic inflammatory cell infiltrate filling the whole thickness of the dermis. The overlying epidermis is normal.

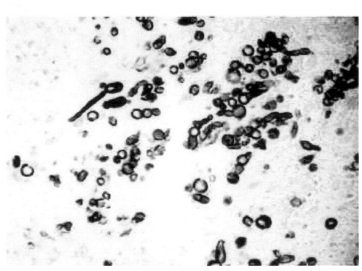

Figure 24c

Phaeohyphomycosis.
Skin histopathology (Grocott stain, high power). There are numerous fungal yeast forms and some short hyphae.

Investigations

Skin histopathology: Biopsy of the lesion revealed a florid granulomatous response in the dermis surrounding numerous fungi. The majority of the fungal structures were yeast-like, but short hyphal structures were also present (Figures 24b, c).

Tissue culture: Culture of tissue on Sabouraud's dextrose agar at 30°C demon-strated growth by colonies characterized by grey and green concentric rings. An isolate was identified as *Alternaria alternata* (Figure 24d).

Diagnosis

Phaeohyphomycosis due to *Alternaria alternata*.

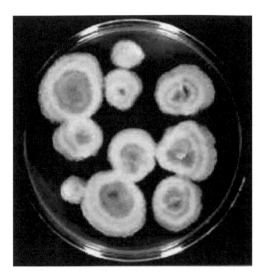

Figure 24d

Phaeohyphomycosis.
Culture of biopsy material showing
multiple cream-coloured colonies
containing concentric green–grey rings
indicative of *Alternaria alternata*.

Treatment and progress

The lesion was debulked surgically and the
patient commenced on itraconazole, initially
at a dose of 200 mg twice daily and then
reduced to 200 mg once daily. Concurrently
his dose of tacrolimus was reduced in view
of an interaction between this drug and
itraconazole. Itraconazole was continued for
a total of 6 months, with complete clearance
of the lesion. There has been no evidence of
recurrence 5 years after treatment.

Comment

Phaeohyphomycosis is a localized cutaneous
infection caused by dematiaceous (pigmented) fungi. A large number of organisms
are implicated in the aetiology of phaeohyphomycosis, including *Alternaria* spp. Many
of the pathogens are found in soil or decom-
posing plant debris. Human infection follows
the traumatic implantation of the fungus
into subcutaneous tissue. Minor trauma
from a thorn or, as in our patient, a wooden
splinter is often sufficient. In a susceptible
host the fungus proliferates to yield a firm
nodule or cystic lesion.

The histology of phaeohyphomycosis often
demonstrates beaded or moniliform hyphae,
and sections through these structures may
give the appearance of yeast-like organisms.
The causative fungi vary in the degree of
pigmentation formed in vivo and it may be
necessary to use Fontana–Masson stain to
demonstrate the pigment in the fungal
cells.

At present, about 80 species of *Alternaria*
have been described, but only eight have
been involved in human or animal infections. *A. alternata* and *A. tenuissima* are the
species most often implicated in cutaneous
alternariosis. Visualization of *Alternaria*
fungi within a skin specimen should be
confirmed by culture and microscopy.
Identification of different species is based on
the conidial morphology.

Immunosuppression appears to be important in the development of cutaneous
alternariosis, and infections have been
described in patients with AIDS, Cushing's
syndrome, lymphoproliferative disorders and
transplant recipients receiving immunosuppressive therapy. The spectrum of clinical
presentation is broad, and cases of verrucous,
eczematous, and ulcerating skin lesions have
all been documented in the literature.

Alternaria spp. are sensitive to imidazole
anti-fungal agents and successful treatment
of cutaneous alternariosis can be achieved
with prolonged administration of itraconazole. In large lesions initial surgical excision
is often recommended as an adjunct to anti-
fungal chemotherapy.

Learning points

1. In the immunosuppressed, minor trauma may result in implantation of organisms not usually pathogenic in immunocompetent individuals.
2. Phaeohyphomycosis is a localized skin infection by pigmented fungi.
3. In a suspected opportunistic skin infection samples must be sent for fungal culture and bacterial culture, as well as routine histopathology.

Reference

Acland KM, Hay RJ, Groves R. Cutaneous infection with *Alternaria alternata* complicating immunosuppression: successful treatment with itraconazole. *Br J Dermatol* 1998; 138: 354–6.

See also case numbers **3, 10, 14, 33.**

Case 25
Photosensitivity with scarring

History

The patient presented at the age of 6 months when his parents noticed the development of painful blisters on the skin of his face and backs of hands following summer sunlight exposure. Blistering was accompanied by increased skin fragility and frequent superficial skin infections. Early in infancy, his urine was noted to be red-brown. By the age of 2 years he was found to have a haemolytic anaemia, which necessitated frequent blood transfusions. Increasing transfusion dependence led to splenomegaly requiring a splenectomy at the age of 6 years. By the age of 17 years, frequent blistering of the facial skin had resulted in significant disfigurement.

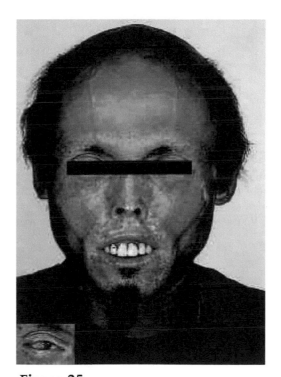

Figure 25a

Congenital erythropoietic porphyria.
There is scarring of the face with retraction of the upper lip and erosions on the lower lip. Photomutilation has shortened the nasal tip. The lateral half of the eyebrows have been lost through scarring. *Insert:* There is corneal scarring secondary to light-induced chronic keratitis.

Clinical features

Examination of the face revealed scarring of the lips with loss of the normal contour of the mouth (Figure 25a). Similar changes had caused foreshortening of the nose and destruction of the ears. The scalp displayed features of an extensive scarring alopecia (Figure 25b). There was hypertrichosis of the hands while cicatrizing changes had resulted in resorption of the terminal digits (Figure 25c). The exposed skin was hyperpigmented.

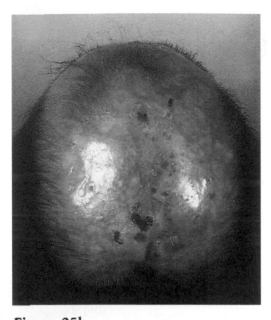

Figure 25b

Congenital erythropoietic porphyria.
There is scarring alopecia and widespread
hair loss. An intact blister and erosions
are visible on the vertex.

The right eye displayed the changes of a
chronic ulcerative keratitis (Figure 25a,
insert). The teeth were discoloured and
fluoresced pink under Wood's light (Figure
25d). The covered skin of the proximal arms,
legs and trunk was normal.

Investigations

Serum uroporphyrin I: 449 000 nmol/24 hr
(normal: <40 nmol/24 hr).

Coproporphyrin I: 133 000 nmol/24 hr
(normal: <280 nmol/24 hr).

Uroporphyrin III and coproporphyrin III: not
detected.

Red cell uroporphyrinogen III synthase activity: 110 nmol uroporphyrinogen III/ml red
cells/hr (normal: 159–352 nmol uroporphyrinogen III/ml red cells/hr).

Diagnosis

**Congenital erythropoietic porphyria (Gunther's
disease).**

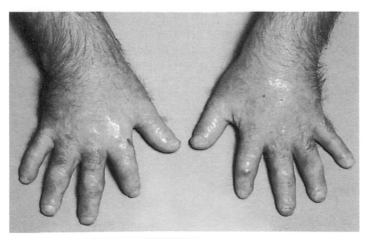

Figure 25c

Congenital erythropoietic porphyria.
Foreshortening of all the digits on the
hands has occurred secondary to bony
resorption of the terminal phalanges.
The skin also displays
hyperpigmentation, hirsutism and the
presence of milia.

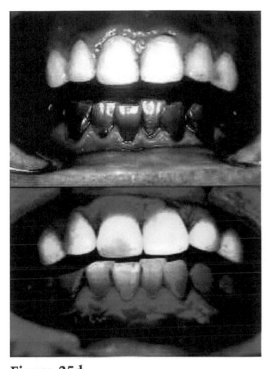

Figure 25d

Congenital erythropoietic porphyria.
Upper panel: The upper teeth have been
capped, the lower teeth are stained dark
by porphyrin deposition. *Lower panel:*
Under Wood's light the lower teeth and
gingivae fluoresce pink due to the presence
of porphyrins.

Progress and treatment

Continued haemolytic anaemia has led to
marrow hyperplasia and generalized reduced
bone density. The need for repeated transfusions has resulted in iron overload despite
treatment with desferrioxamine, which is
administered continuously via a syringe
driver. The patient developed acute hepatitis
at the age of 28 and was found to be hepatitis B positive. A liver biopsy at that time
showed grade 4 siderosis with portal inflammation, fibrosis and bridging.

The patient uses Dundee sunscreen (which
provides some photoprotection at wave-
lengths above 400 nm). Despite this, he still
develops cutaneous blistering after 15
minutes of light exposure between the
months of February and November. For
many years the patient received high-dose
beta-carotene but without appreciable reduction in photosensitivity.

Despite these problems, our patient has
continued to work and, although he restricts
his exposure to summer sunlight, he leads as
normal a life as possible.

Comment

Congenital erythropoietic porphyria (CEP) or
Gunther's disease is an extremely rare
autosomal recessive disorder of haem biosyn-
thesis caused by a deficiency of the enzyme
uroporphyrinogen III synthase. This metabolic defect leads to an accumulation of
porphyrinogens, which are in turn converted
into photoactive porphyrins. Porphyrins in
the skin absorb light of wavelength around
410 nm. The resulting phototoxic reaction
causes blistering, which is responsible for
photomutilation of exposed skin. The severity of the photosensitivity encountered in
CEP often leads affected patients to shun
sunlight completely.

The accumulation of porphyrins induces
chronic haemolysis, which results in
splenomegaly and reactive erythroid hyperplasia, the latter predisposing to bone
fragility. The cause of the haemolytic
anaemia in these patients is unknown.
Proposed mechanisms include photohaemol-
ysis in the superficial circulation or an
associated red cell defect perhaps exacerbated
by high levels of circulating porphyrins.
Hypertransfusion has been reported to
control the photosensitivity of CEP and
reduce porphyrin production in about 50% of

patients by the suppression of erythropoiesis. However, the level of transfusion required to maintain a haematocrit of over 35% can lead to problems with excessive iron overload, as in our patient. Severe iron overload can lead to the development of siderosis, which, if left untreated, may result in progressive liver failure.

The overall management of CEP has centred on attempts at decreasing porphyrin overproduction and reducing porphyrin absorption within the gastrointestinal tract by interruption of the enterohepatic circulation. Recently, allogeneic haematopoietic stem cell transplantation from identical HLA-matched siblings has been used successfully, with, in some cases, resolution of haemolysis and photosensitivity.

Reference

Desnick RJ, Astrin KH. Congenital erythropoietic porphyria: advances in pathogenesis and treatment. *Br J Haematol* 2002; 117: 779–95.

See also case number 16.

Case 26
Swelling of the hands and generalized hyperpigmentation

History

A 54-year-old West Indian woman was referred with a 2-year history of generalized darkening of her skin. The pigmentary changes were accompanied by pruritus, especially of the arms and legs. She had also noticed swelling of the hands and fingers. On closer questioning, she admitted to increasing fatigue, myalgia of the arms and legs, and sub-sternal discomfort on eating. She gave a long history of Raynaud's phenomenon with typical triphasic changes.

Clinical findings

Large areas of macular hyperpigmentation were present on her upper back, abdomen, arms, legs and face (Figure 26a). On her torso and limbs there were, additionally, small well-circumscribed areas of depigmentation. The hands and fingers were swollen, the skin being tight and indurated (Figure 26b). The cuticles of all finger nails were irregular and ragged while examination of the proximal nail folds revealed visible, dilated capillary loops (Figure 26c).

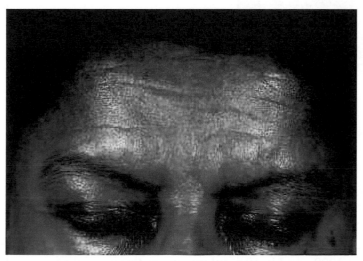

Figure 26a

Scleroderma.
The patient presented with widespread increased pigmentation. There is hyperpigmentation on the forehead; her normal colouring is the brown of the glabellar skin.

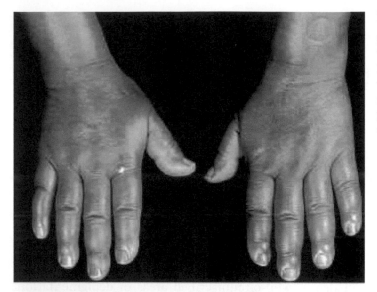

Figure 26b

Scleroderma.
The fingers and hands are swollen.
Note the impression made by the
watch strap at the left wrist. The skin
is tight and shiny. There is a small
patch of depigmentation on the dorsal
aspect of the right hand.

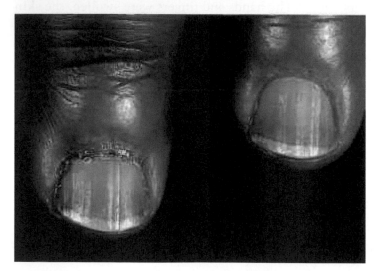

Figure 26c

Scleroderma.
The tips of the fingers are swollen.
The cuticle of the middle finger (on
left) is ragged and there are visible
capillaries in the proximal nail fold.

Investigations

FBC: normal, U&E: normal, LFT: normal,
CPK: normal. ESR: 40 mm/1st hr.

ANA: 1:40, double-stranded DNA antibodies:
negative, RF: negative.

ENA, including Ro, La, Sm, RNP, Jo-1 and
Scl-70: all negative.

Anti-centromere antibody: positive >1:1000.

Oesphageal scinitigraphy: severe dysmotility.

Echocardiography: There was evidence of
pulmonary hypertension, but good left
ventricular function.

Diagnosis

Limited cutaneous systemic sclerosis.

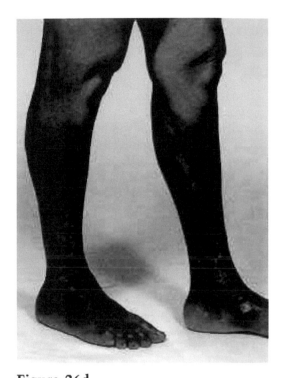

Figure 26d

Scleroderma.
Sclerotic changes of the lower legs with
hyperpigmentation and 'waisting' of the
gaiter skin. There is an ulcer on the dorsal
aspect of the left foot.

Treatment and progress

Over 12 years of follow-up the patient has
developed cutaneous sclerosis with sclerodactyly of the fingers. Involvement of the
feet and lower legs has also produced
sclerotic changes and chronic ulceration
(Figure 26d). Telangiectasiae have appeared
on the finger tips and lips. The skin of the
face and trunk remains hyperpigmented and
continues to be itchy. Her exertional
dyspnoea has worsened, reflecting pulmonary hypertension. Oesophagitis and
gastroparesis continue to induce retrosternal
chest pain.

Treatments that have been used, with
minimal benefit include prednisolone, methylprednisolone, methotrexate, azathioprine and
mycophenolate mofetil. Currently, the patient
is receiving nifedipine for the Raynaud's
phenomenon, and omeprazole and cisapride to
help reduce the effects of oesophageal
dysmotility.

Comment

Systemic sclerosis (SS) is characterized by
fibrosis of skin and internal organs as well as
widespread damage to small blood vessels.
The hallmark of the disease is scleroderma
typified by tight, indurated, thickened skin.
Scleroderma associated with internal
involvement is divided into limited
cutaneous SS and diffuse cutaneous SS.

Limited cutaneous SS, previously known as
CREST syndrome (Calcinosis, Raynaud's,
oEsophageal dysmotility, Scleroderma, Telangiectases), is associated with anti-
centromere antibodies in approximately 80%
of patients. Affected individuals are usually
female, aged 30–50 years, and commonly
have a long history of Raynaud's phenomenon. Skin changes are most marked on the
limbs and face, with less prominent involvement of the trunk. A common presentation
is with swelling of the hands and fingers,
often with localized pain, which can be
mistaken for carpal tunnel syndrome. In
black skin, early scleroderma frequently
causes pigmentary changes, both hyperpigmentation and hypopigmentation, as seen in
our patient. Visible, dilated nail fold capillary
loops are common, as is the presence of
digital and facial telangiectasiae. Long-stand-

ing disease involvement of the mouth results in microstomia. Finger tip skin ulceration can be caused by cutaneous ischaemia and by the extrusion of calcinotic lesions. The major long-term complications of limited cutaneous SS are malabsorption from small intestinal involvement and right-sided heart failure secondary to pulmonary hypertension.

In contrast, diffuse cutaneous SS is characterized by more widespread skin changes with truncal as well as acral scleroderma: 30% of patients with diffuse cutaneous SS possess anti-topoisomerase 1 (Scl-70) antibodies. There is an early and significant incidence of interstitial lung disease, oliguric renal failure, diffuse gastrointestinal disease and myocardial involvement.

Scleroderma is a chronic disease that is difficult to manage. Treatment should be directed to improve Raynaud's phenomenon, to modify immunological damage and to treat specific organ problems. For the skin involvement, general management with emollients can be helpful, while appropriate dressings and surgical measures should be employed for managing ulceration and calcinosis.

Learning points

1. In black skin systemic sclerosis (SS) can present with pigmentary skin changes, both hyperpigmentation and hypopigmentation.
2. Swelling of the hands and fingers with a history of Raynaud's phenomenon should suggest a diagnosis of SS.
3. Limited cutaneous SS is characterized by prominent acral involvement, a positive anti-centromere antibody and a better prognosis than diffuse cutaneous SS.

Reference

Foeldvari I. Diffuse and limited cutaneous systemic scleroderma. *Curr Opin Rheumatol* 2000; 12: 435–8.

See also case numbers 7, 21, 46.

Case 27
Birthmarks and macrodactyly

History

A 24-year-old woman presented with a transient inflammatory dermatosis that had resolved by the time of her consultation. Despite this, a full examination was undertaken and it was found that she had a number of congenital cutaneous abnormalities and bony anomalies. The patient was born of healthy, unrelated parents. At birth, she was noticed to have large feet, which subsequently grew rapidly. The feet were markedly deformed, with cerebriform hypertrophy of the skin. Multiple corrective orthopaedic operations were performed during her childhood. However, at the age of 9 years she underwent bilateral forefoot amputations. In the past, she had been diagnosed initially as having neurofibromatosis, but subsequently her cutaneous features were thought to be more in keeping with Kippel–Trenaunay syndrome.

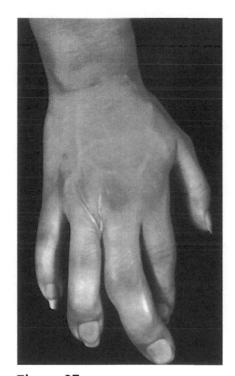

Figure 27a

Proteus syndrome.
There is macrodactyly with enlarged, curving fingers. This is the immediate clue to the diagnosis.

Clinical findings

The fingers of her right hand were abnormally large and curved (Figure 27a). Further cutaneous examination revealed a warty lymphangiomatous lesion on her left chest wall and a large pigmented macule on the lower abdomen that extended to the midline

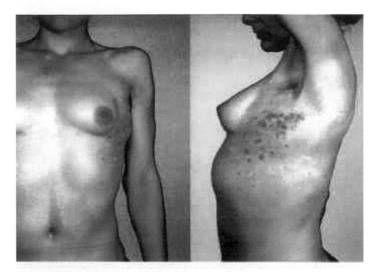

Figure 27b

Proteus syndrome.
Various forms of naevi accompany the
disorder. An extensive lymphangioma
circumscriptum involves the left
upper lateral chest. There is also
naevoid hyperpigmentation present on
the left lower abdominal skin
following Blaschko's lines and
showing a sharp cut-off at the
midline.

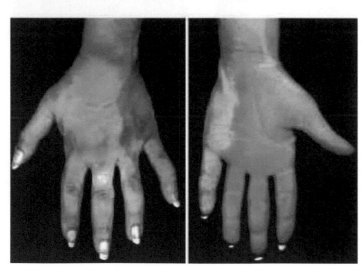

Figure 27c

Proteus syndrome.
There is an epidermal naevus
covering most of the left palm and
wrist.

(Figure 27b). There was a lesion on her left
shoulder, consistent with a verrucous epidermal naevus that extended onto the arm and
hand following Blaschko's lines (Figure 27c).
She also had prominent venous varicosities
affecting the left arm and scattered lipomas.

Investigations

Skin histopathology of chest lesion:
lymphangioma circumscriptum.

Skin histopathology of dorsal foot skin:
There was an acanthotic and hyperkeratotic
epidermis, with a plexiform mass of nerve
fascicles in the subcutaneous fat.

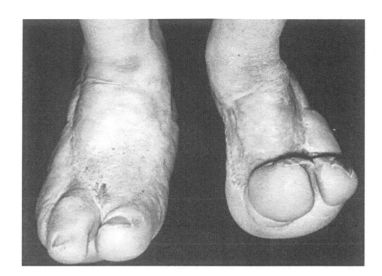

Figure 27d

Proteus syndrome.
This photograph was taken of the patient's feet at the age of 9 years, prior to bilateral forefoot amputation. There is macrodactyly and evidence of previous surgery.

Diagnosis

Proteus syndrome.

Treatment and progress

The patient was unconcerned about the presence of the naevi. No orthopaedic intervention was offered for the skeletal abnormalities.

Comment

Proteus syndrome is named after the Greek god Proteus ('the old man of the sea'), who had the power to appear in the form of any creature he wished. He knew everything in the past, present and future, but hated to divulge the information and therefore changed his shape at will to avoid capture. The protean manifestations of this disorder result from congenital hamartomas causing cutaneous and skeletal overgrowth.

A broad range of clinical features may be present and some individuals are more severely affected than others. Skeletal and soft tissue overgrowth can involve any part of the body, resulting in partial gigantism of hands or feet and other forms of hemihypertrophy, including macrocephaly. Macrodactyly is particularly characteristic, with distinctive cerebriform overgrowth of the plantar or palmar soft tissues. A number of different cutaneous lesions also occur, including epidermal naevi, vascular naevi (port-wine stains, angiomas, cavernous lymphangiomas and lymphangioma circumscriptum) and soft tissue masses, particularly lipomas. Areas of macular hypo- or hyperpigmentation have been reported.

Non-cutaneous findings include skeletal abnormalities, ocular problems, learning difficulties and epilepsy.

Recent genetic analysis of individuals with Proteus syndrome have identified germline mutations in the *PTEN* tumour suppressor gene. Originally shown to be a major susceptibility gene for Cowden syndrome (characterized by facial tricholemmonas, multiple oral fibromatous papules and an increased risk of breast and thyroid cancers) the PTEN hamartoma tumour syndrome has broadened to include Proteus syndrome and other related disorders. PTEN is a protein phosphatase that mediates growth suppression via the PI3-kinase/AKT pro-apoptotic pathway. Disruption of PTEN-mediated apoptosis, as in Proteus syndrome, appears to permit uncontrolled hamartomatous tissue overgrowth.

To make the diagnosis of Proteus syndrome a scoring system has been developed: 13 or more points are required to establish the diagnosis. Our patient scored 17 points.

Proteus syndrome scoring system

Feature	Score
Macrodactyly and/or hemihypertrophy	5
Plantar and/or palmar cerebriform hyperplasia	4
Lipomas and subcutaneous tumours	4
Verrucous epidermal naevus	3
Macrocephaly or skull exostoses	2.5
Miscellaneous minor abnormalities	1

Before Proteus syndrome was described in 1983, many patients were thought to have other congenital hamartomatous disorders, such as Kippel–Trenaunay syndrome (venous varicosities, port-wine stains and limb hypertrophy), Bannayan–Zonana syndrome (macrodactyly, subcutaneous lipomatosis and megalencephaly) and Maffucci's syndrome (macrodactyly, limb hyperpertrophy and asymmetry and enchondromas). Joseph Merrick, the Elephant Man, is now thought to have suffered from Proteus syndrome; he

had macrocephaly, skull hyperostoses, long bone hypertrophy, and thickened skin and subcutaneous tissues. In the past he was labelled as having neurofibromatosis, but there was no family history, no reports of café-au-lait patches and no histological evidence of neurofibromas.

The aim of treatment in Proteus syndrome is to limit disability. Contributions can be made by plastic and orthopaedic surgeons and physiotherapists. However, despite treatment, the disorder may be responsible for marked degrees of deformity.

Learning points

1. Conduct a thorough examination on all patients. You never know what you may find!
2. Proteus syndrome results from multiple congenital hamartomas causing skeletal, soft tissue and cutaneous lesions.
3. Proteus syndrome and Cowden syndrome are both caused by mutations in the *PTEN* tumour suppressor gene.

Reference

Waite KA, Eng C. Protean PTEN: form and function. *Am J Hum Genet* 2002; 70: 829–44.

See also case number 48.

Case 28
Facial nodules, cough and breathlessness

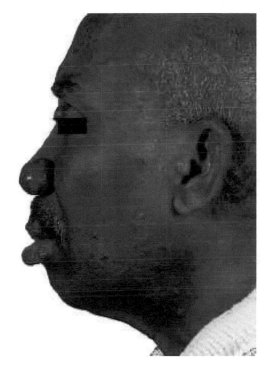

History

A 55-year-old Jamaican nightclub singer presented with a 2-month history of rapidly enlarging facial nodules. In addition, he complained of cough, breathlessness and red, sore eyes. He had lost 4 kg in weight over the past 3 months.

Clinical findings

There were numerous red-brown papules and nodules on his face located predominantly on the eyelids, lips, jaw and ears (Figure 28a). Auscultation of his chest revealed crepitations at the bases and mid zones. Slit-lamp examination demonstrated bilateral anterior uveitis.

Figure 28a

Sarcoidosis.
There are multiple red-brown papules and nodules involving the eyelids, nose, lips, jaw and ears.

Investigations

Hb: 10.3 g/dl (11.5–15.5 g/dl), WCC: 6.9 × 10^9/l (4.0–11.0 × 10^9/l), plts 447 × 10^9/l (150–450 × 10^9/l). ESR 42 mm/hr (1–10 mm/hr).

U&E: normal, LFT: normal, calcium: 2.63 mmol/l (2.20–2.60 mmol/l), serum ACE: 93 U/I (8–52 U/I).

Chest x-ray: bilateral hilar lymphadenopathy (Figure 28b).

Skin histopathology: Biopsy of a facial nodule demonstrated intense dermal inflammation characterized by aggregates of epithelioid cells forming discrete, lymphocyte-poor, non-caseating granulomas. Multinucleate giant cells were also present (Figure 28c).

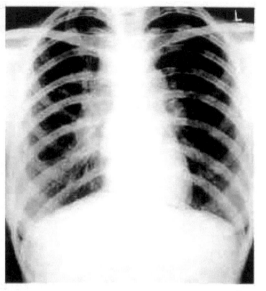

Figure 28b

Sarcoidosis.
Chest x-ray showing bilateral hilar lymphadenopathy.

Diagnosis

Sarcoidosis.

Treatment and progress

The patient was commenced on prednisolone 30 mg daily, which rapidly controlled his respiratory, ocular and cutaneous symptoms. However, the patient developed steroid-induced diabetes necessitating reduction in prednisolone, which in turn resulted in recurrence of the cutaneous lesions. Mepacrine was added at a dose of 100 mg twice daily, which induced good clearance of the cutaneous lesions but was accompanied by hyperpigmentation (Figure 28d). At 3-year follow-up the cutaneous and systemic sarcoid remained controlled on prednisolone 7.5 mg once daily and mepacrine 100 mg taken on alternate days.

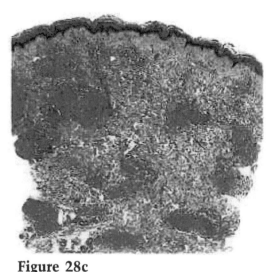

Figure 28c

Sarcoidosis.
Skin histopathology (H&E, low power). Well-circumscribed, epithelioid, lymphocyte-poor granulomas are present throughout the dermis.

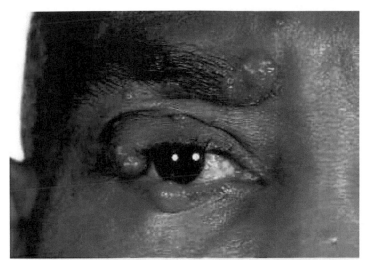

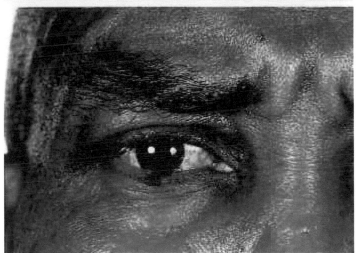

Figure 28d

Sarcoidosis.
Upper panel: Before treatment there were large nodules involving the eyebrows and eyelids. *Lower panel:* After treatment with prednisolone and mepacrine the skin lesions have completely resolved. Note the hyperpigmentation secondary to the use of mepacrine.

Comment

Sarcoidosis affects all races, both sexes and all ages. There are two peaks of onset: one between the ages of 15 and 35 years, and a second in women aged 45–65 years. In African and West Indian patients sarcoidosis has a tendency to be more severe than in other races.

Sarcoidosis is a multi-system disorder and the sites of involvement in any given patient will determine the presentation and morbid-

ity. On average, 25% of sarcoidosis cases have cutaneous involvement, which can occur at any stage. As in our case, skin lesions often develop early and it is not unusual for the dermatologist to make the diagnosis of sarcoidosis.

Sarcoidosis skin lesions can classified as specific if they contain granulomas and non-specific if the pathology is reactive. Common specific sarcoidosis skin lesions are papules, nodules, plaques, subcutaneous nodules, infiltrative scars, and lupus pernio.

Uncommon presentations include annular, ulcerative, psoriasiform, hypopigmented and verrucous lesions. Other manifestations of skin sarcoidosis are ichthyosis, cicatricial alopecia, erythroderma and unilateral limb oedema. The non-specific lesion that is strongly associated with sarcoidosis is erythema nodosum. In general, specific skin lesions have no prognostic significance; however, the presence of erythema nodosum is associated with sarcoidosis that resolves spontaneously.

Corticosteroids are the cornerstone of therapy in sarcoidosis: non-oral therapy for limited cutaneous disease includes superpotent topical corticosteroids and intralesional triamcinolone. Carbon dioxide or pulsed dye laser can be successful in treating lupus pernio. Oral corticosteroids are indicated in extensive cutaneous sarcoidosis and with significant systemic involvement. Antimalarial drugs, such as hydroxychloroquine and mepacrine, can be used as steroid-sparing agents. Other second-line drugs shown to have efficacy in sarcoidosis include methotrexate, retinoids, tetracyclines and thalidomide.

Learning points

1. Sarcoidosis commonly presents with skin signs, either specific granulomatous lesions or erythema nodosum.
2. A biopsy of specific skin lesions is the easiest method of obtaining tissue for diagnosis. Histopathology will demonstrate lymphocyte-poor, non-caseating granulomas.
3. Although corticosteroids are first-line therapy, anti-malarial drugs can be useful as steroid-sparing agents.

Reference

Mana J, Marcoval J, Graells J et al. Cutaneous involvement in sarcoidosis: relation to systemic disease. *Arch Dermatol* 1997; 133: 882–8.

See also case numbers 3 and 11.

Case 29
A unilateral breast rash

History

A 43-year-old woman was referred with an eruption involving the skin of the left breast. Two years previously she had undergone a wide local excision of an invasive ductal carcinoma of the left breast and clearance of the axilla, which had yielded negative lymph nodes. She subsequently received adjuvant chemotherapy and radical radiotherapy to the left breast. Three months prior to presentation she had noticed the development of a rash involving the left areola. An initial skin biopsy was inconclusive; however, the dermatosis extended and she was therefore referred to the dermatology department.

Clinical findings

Examination revealed an erythematous eruption involving the areola and skin of the medial aspect of the left breast (Figure 29a). The lesional skin was warm and indurated with multiple palpable dermal nodules (Figure 29b).

Investigations

Skin histology: Biopsy of lesional skin revealed diffuse infiltration of the full thickness

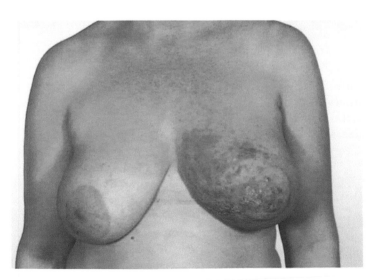

Figure 29a

Carcinoma erysipeloides.
There is an an erythematous eruption involving the skin of the medial side of the left breast.

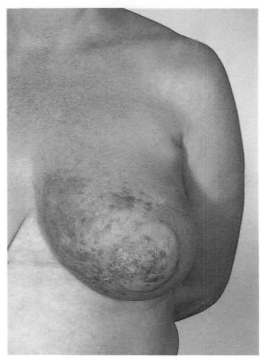

Figure 29b

Carcinoma erysipeloides.
The lesional skin was red, warm and
indurated.

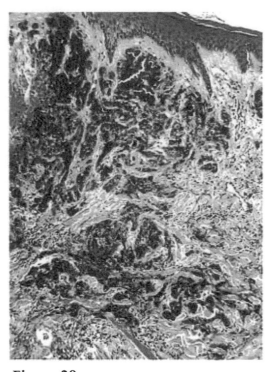

Figure 29c

Carcinoma erysipeloides.
Skin histopathology (H&E, medium
power). There is invasive carcinoma
within the dermis showing cellular
pleomorphism, acinar formation and, in
places, necrosis.

of the dermis by poorly differentiated adenocarcinoma. The neoplastic tissue demonstrated similar features to the invasive ductal
carcinoma observed in the original breast
biopsy (Figure 29c).

Diagnosis

Carcinoma erysipeloides.

Treatment and progress

The patient underwent further investigations
to search for other possible sites of metastasis. A liver ultrasound scan, chest x-ray and
bone scan were normal. The patient received
chemotherapy and radiotherapy and thereafter underwent a left mastectomy, the
defect being resurfaced with latissimus dorsi
muscle and an overlying split skin graft.

Five months later she was noted to have a
rash involving the right nipple. A biopsy
confirmed further intracutaneous carcinoma.

She underwent a right mastectomy, which demonstrated grade III ductal carcinoma infiltrating the breast and involving regional lymph nodes. Thereafter she received radical radiotherapy to the right chest wall.

Comment

Carcinoma erysipeloides (CE) is a form of cutaneous metastatic adenocarcinoma in which there is intralymphatic spread, usually from a breast carcinoma, to the overlying skin. The name reflects the clinical appearance of an erysipelas-like eruption characterized by a well-defined area of warm, indurated erythema. The redness appears to be a consequence of dermal lymphatic involvement with tumour, while vasodilatation is further enhanced by the local release of vasoactive cytokines. Histologically, there is lymphatic plugging with adenocarcinoma at all levels of the dermis. Clinically, CE complicating breast cancer presents as rapidly evolving unilateral anterior chest wall erythema, which may extend to the back, involve the proximal arm and even cross the midline.

CE is one of several manifestations of lymphatic spread of breast cancer to the anterior chest wall skin. Nodular carcinoma is characterized by multiple, firm erythematous nodules of varying size. Carcinoma telangiectaticum occurs when there is prominent obstruction of the small blood vessels of the upper dermis producing sclerotic, telangiectatic plaques. In carcinoma *en cuirasse*, there is non-inflammatory cutaneous induration resulting from diffuse infiltration of tumour cells between dermal collagen bundles and associated reactive fibrosis.

Although there are reports of patients who have survived many years after the appearance of cutaneous metastases, dissemination to the skin is usually indicative of advanced cancer spread and poor prognosis.

Learning points

1. In a patient with a history of breast cancer a rash on the breast should be biopsied to exclude carcinoma erysipeloides or another form of cutaneous metastasis.
2. Cutaneous metastatic disease in breast cancer can present with cellulitic, telangiectatic or sclerotic skin changes.
3. Cutaneous metastases usually indicate a poor prognosis.

Reference

Cox SE, Cruz PD Jr. A spectrum of inflammatory metastasis to the skin via lymphatics: three cases of carcinoma erysipeloides. *J Am Acad Dermatol* 1994; 30: 304–7.

See also case number 36.

Case 30
Fever and a desquamating rash in an infant

History

A 4-month-old baby girl presented with a 7-day history of a fever, rash and vomiting. The child had been born prematurely at 31 weeks and had spent 6 weeks on the special care baby unit. She had been admitted 2 months earlier with an episode of bronchiolitis.

Clinical findings

The child was febrile (40°C). There was a widespread scarlatiniform erythema of the trunk, limbs and face as well as palmo-plantar erythema (Figures 30a). Involvement of the nappy area was severe with extensive desquamation. The lips were red and inflamed. The heart rate was 180 beats per minute. Auscultation revealed an ejection systolic murmur at the left sternal edge radiating through to the back. There was cervical lymphadenopathy.

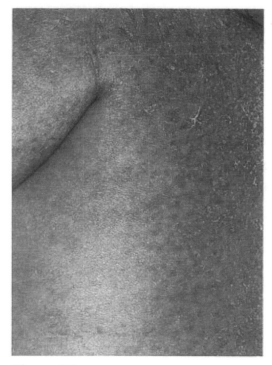

Figure 30a

Kawasaki disease.
There is a scarlatinaform erythema with fine scaling and desquamation which had followed a high persistent fever.

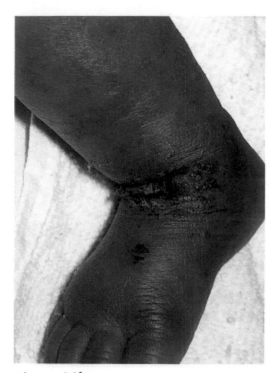

Figure 30b

Kawasaki disease.
Desquamation of the right foot occurring
late in the course of this disease.

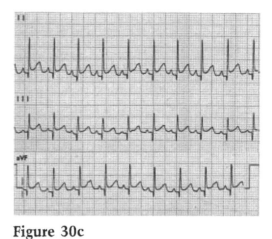

Figure 30c

Kawasaki disease.
ECG demonstrating Q waves in the
inferior leads (II, III, aVF), indicating
myocardial ischaemia.

Investigations

Hb: 8.3 g/dl (11.5–15.5 g/dl), WCC: 28 × 10^9/l
(4.0–11.0 × 10^9/l), PMN: 20.3 × 10^9/l (2.0–7.5
× 10^9/l), plts: 969 × 10^9/l (150–450 × 10^9/l).
ESR: 120 mm/hr (1–10 mm/hr).

ECG: sinus tachycardia, Q waves in leads II,
III and aVF (Figure 30c).

Echocardiography (performed 12 days after
admission): This showed a structurally normal
heart with normal ventricular function and no
evidence of dyskinesia. However, there was
marked aneurysmal dilatation of the left
mainstem, circumflex and left anterior
descending coronary arteries, together with
less marked dilatation of right coronary artery.

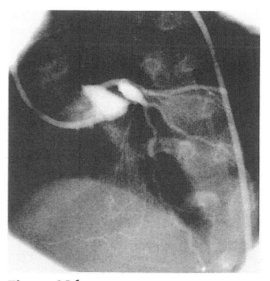

Figure 30d

Kawasaki disease.
Coronary angiography reveals two
aneurysms in the left mainstem artery.

Diagnosis

Kawasaki disease.

Treatment and progress

The patient was commenced on high-dose aspirin (100 mg/kg/day in 4 divided doses) and intravenous immunoglobulin (2 g/kg infused over 12 hours). The inflammatory rash settled in the groins, but desquamation of the trunk and peeling of the palmo-plantar skin occurred subsequently (Figure 30b). Two weeks after the initiation of treatment the erythrocyte sedimentation rate (ESR) and platelet count had dropped significantly. She was converted to low-dose aspirin after 1 month of treatment and discharged from hospital. At this stage, a coronary angiogram demonstrated persistent aneurysms of both left and right coronary arteries (Figure 30d). Low-dose aspirin was continued for a further year, by which time echocardiography revealed resolution of the aneurysms.

Comment

Kawasaki disease (mucocutaneous lymph node syndrome) is a multi-system disorder occurring in young children and characterized by a widespread, occasionally fatal, vasculitis. It is generally believed that Kawasaki disease is caused by an infectious agent in a genetically susceptible individual which results in an abnormal host reaction. The evidence for an infectious cause includes the identification of geographical clustering, an increased incidence among siblings and the predominance amongst young children.

A high persistent fever is often the presenting feature and is followed by a variety of mucocutaneous changes, including erythema of palmo-plantar skin, swelling of the hands and feet, lymphadenopathy, and injection of the conjunctival and oropharyngeal mucosae. The dermatosis is particularly prominent in the nappy area, where there is marked erythema and early desquamation. Exanthems associated with Kawasaki disease are variable and include scarlatiniform eruptions, erythroderma and erythema multiforme. In the convalescent stage a distinctive pattern of acral desquamation occurs, beginning at the tips of the fingers and progressing proximally. Although there is no specific diagnostic test for Kawasaki disease, a characteristic finding is marked thrombocytosis, which is usually present by week 2 of the illness. Other less specific haematological abnormalities include mild anaemia, elevated ESR, and leucocytosis. Skin biopsy findings from the exanthems of Kawasaki disease are non-specific and do not usually demonstrate vasculitis.

Cardiovascular complications are the most significant determinants of long-term morbidity and mortality, and therefore repeated examination and investigation of the cardiovascular system is mandatory. Abnormalities include cardiac murmurs, cardiomegaly, ECG abnormalities (prolonged PR and QT intervals, abnormal Q waves, ST changes and arrythmias), myocarditis, valvular insufficiency and, most notably, coronary artery aneurysms, which occur in 10–20% of untreated patients.

Intravenous immunoglobulin plus high-dose aspirin have been effective in reducing the incidence and severity of the coronary artery abnormalities. The risk is reduced to 3% if therapy is given in the first 10 days of the illness. Aspirin is discontinued after 6 weeks of treatment if repeated echocardiography is normal and the ESR and platelet count are normal. If coronary artery aneurysms are persistent, low-dose aspirin is continued and should be administered for 1 year after the aneurysms have resolved on echocardiography.

Learning points

1. Kawasaki disease must be considered in a sick infant with a high persistent fever, palmo-plantar erythema and a desquamating flexural rash.
2. Life-threatening cardiovascular complications, secondary to coronary artery aneurysms, can develop if the diagnosis is missed and treatment delayed. Early investigation with echocardiography is mandatory.
3. Treatment with high-dose aspirin and intravenous immunoglobulin can reduce the incidence and severity of coronary artery disease

Reference

Brogan PA, Bose A, Burgner D et al. Kawasaki disease: an evidence based approach to diagnosis, treatment and proposals for future research. *Arch Dis Child* 2002; 86: 286–90.

See also case number 15.

Case 31
A follicular eruption in a vegan

History

A 22-year-old woman presented with a 3-month history of a rash, particularly affecting her arms and legs. On direct questioning it emerged that she had been a strict vegan from the age of 5 years, influenced by a teacher who declaimed against eating meat. Her basic daily diet consisted of potatoes and biscuits. There was no past medical history of note and she was not on any regular medication.

Clinical findings

Examination revealed a pale and underweight young woman with a widespread rash over her trunk and limbs (Figures 31a, b). The eruption was composed of groups of small (1–2 mm) erythematous, hyperkeratotic, perifollicular papules (Figure 31c). Her flexures were spared and there were no abnormalities of nails, hair or scalp.

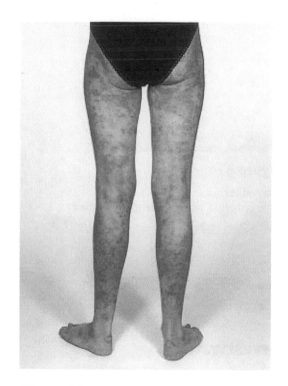

Figure 31a
Phrynoderma.
There is a widespread papular eruption involving the legs.

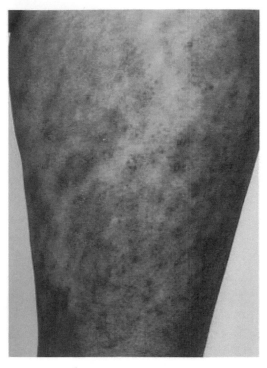

Figure 31b

Phrynoderma.
The eruption consists of perifollicular papules.

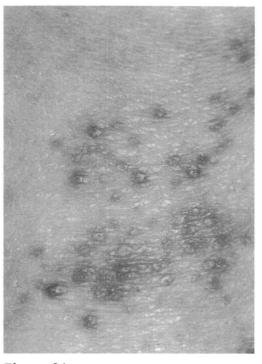

Figure 31c

Phrynoderma.
Some lesions have a central keratin plug.

Investigations

Hb: 10.0 g/dl (11.5–15.5 g/dl), MCV: 135.6 fl (79.0–96.0 fl).

Serum vitamin B_{12}: 45 ng/l (180–1100 ng/l), serum vitamin A: 0.3 µmol/l (0.3–4.5 µmol/l).

Serum zinc: 10.6 µmol/l (10.1–29.7 µmol/l).

Albumin 34 g/l (35–50 g/l).

Other vitamins and essential minerals: normal.

Small bowel permeability studies: normal.

Skin histopathology: Biopsy of a papule revealed discontinuous parakeratosis affecting the follicular epidermis but sparing the non-follicular epidermis. Follicular plugging with keratin was also evident (Figure 31d).

Diagnosis

Phrynoderma.

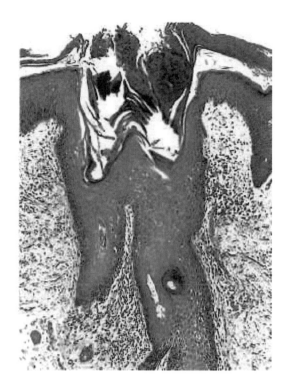

Figure 31d

Phrynoderma.
Histopathology of skin biopsy (H&E, medium power). There is hyperkeratosis and plugging of the dilated follicular orifice, parakeratosis of the follicular epidermis and a folliculocentric chronic inflammatory cell infiltrate.

Treatment and progress

The patient was seen by the dietitians and was commenced on a balanced diet. Her vitamin B_{12} deficiency was replaced with intramuscular hydroxycobalamin 1 mg 3 times per week for 2 weeks. At follow-up 1 month later her eruption had resolved and repeat blood tests were within normal range. She is no longer a vegan.

Comment

The term 'phrynoderma' was coined in 1933 to describe a papular skin eruption observed in malnourished prisoners, the appearance of which closely resembled the skin of a toad (Greek: *phrynos* - toad). Phrynoderma typically consists of perifollicular hyperkeratotic papules. The papules contain a central keratin plug, which may be shed leaving a large crater and be mistaken for a perforating disorder. The lesions typically affect the extensor surfaces but may extend to affect the thighs and arms. The pathological process is one of hyperkeratinization of the epithelium lining the hair follicle, thus producing follicular plugging.

Phrynoderma is a disease of malnutrition and is now rarely seen in developed countries. The dermatological sequelae to malnourishment can be non-specific, such as hyperpigmentation and ichthyosis, or specific due to a lack of individual nutrients. The specific syndromes include scurvy secondary to a lack of vitamin C, and pellagra due to niacin deficiency. The precise deficiency leading to phrynoderma remains in question and a range of nutritional deficiencies have been implicated. However, many papers have suggested that a specific lack of vitamin A induces the follicular hyperkeratinization characteristic of this dermatosis. Our case displayed the typical clinical features of phrynoderma and responded extremely well to correction of her nutritional deficiencies. However, the most notable measured deficiency was of vitamin B_{12}, which would suggest, at least in our patient, a role for a lack of this vitamin in the pathogenesis of phrynoderma.

Learning points

1. In a malnourished or anorexic patient the development of a widespread eruption of perifollicular hyperkeratotic papules should suggest a diagnosis of phrynoderma.
2. Most cases of phrynoderma have been reported in association with vitamin A deficiency; however, lack of other vitamins and essential nutrients has also been implicated.
3. Other dermatoses secondary to malnourishment include scurvy, which is caused by a lack of vitamin C, and pellagra, due to niacin deficiency.

Reference

Nakjang Y, Yuttanavivat T. Phrynoderma: a review of 105 cases. *J Dermatol* 1988; 15: 531–4.

See also case number 12.

Case 32
Erythroderma in a Jamaican man

History

A 48-year-old man from Jamaica presented with an itchy, eczematous dermatosis. The rash initially responded to topical steroids but within 1 year the patient had developed a generalized eruption. Apart from intense pruritus he was otherwise well. He had no past medical history of note.

Clinical findings

On examination, the patient was erythrodermic with an exfoliative dermatitis. There was extensive lichenification with numerous, widespread excoriations. The thickened skin hung in coarse folds on the torso. There was severe palmo–plantar hyperkeratosis. There was lymphadenopathy at the axillae and groins but no hepatosplenomegaly (Figure 32a).

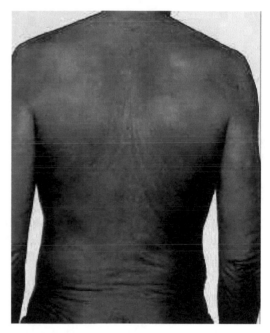

Figure 32a

Erythrodermic adult T-cell leukaemia/lymphoma.
There is erythroderma with diffuse erythema, hyperpigmentation and coarse skin folds of the back and waist.

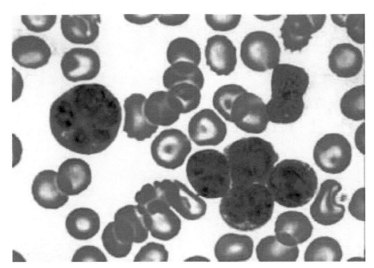

Figure 32b

Adult T-cell leukaemia/lymphoma.
The blood film is characterized by the presence of atypical leucocytes with markedly convoluted and lobulated nuclei with a flower petal configuration (so-called 'flower cells'). These cells have the immunophenotypic characteristics of T cells.

Investigations

Hb: 11.5 g/dl (11.5–15.5 g/dl), WCC 22.7 × 10^9/l (4.0–11.0 × 10^9/l), lymphs: 16 × 10^9/l (1.3–4.0 × 10^9/l)), plts: 376 × 10^9/l (150–450 × 10^9/l).

Blood film: numerous abnormal lymphocytes ('flower cells') (Figure 32b).

Skin histopathology: There was diffuse skin involvement by adult T-cell leukaemia/lymphoma (ATLL) with atypical lymphocytes in the dermis (Figure 32c).

HTLV-1 serology: positive.

Lymph node histology: There was replacement of the normal architecture by an large numbers of atypical lymphocytes bearing the T-cell phenotype (CD3$^+$, CD4$^+$, CD5$^+$).

Total-body CT scan: widespread lymphadenopathy.

Diagnosis

HTLV-1-associated erythrodermic adult T-cell leukaemia/lymphoma.

Treatment and progress

Systemic treatment with acitretin induced a prolonged remission, after which his disease progressed with night sweats, weight loss, refractory erythroderma and intractable pruritus. His skin showed generalized erythema and scaling with palmo–plantar hyperkeratosis and infiltration of the face and scalp. The skin of the latter was longitudinally and irregularly folded to give a cerebriform appearance (cutis verticis gyrata) (Figure 32d). A repeat CT scan revealed hepatosplenomegaly in addition to widespread lymphadenopathy. He received, in turn, UVB phototherapy, interferon-α plus AZT, deoxycoformycin, total-body skin electron-beam radiotherapy, extracorporeal photophoresis and CHOP chemotherapy, all to no benefit. The patient's pruritus and erythroderma

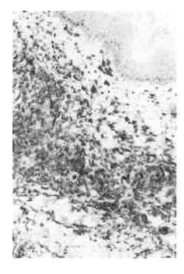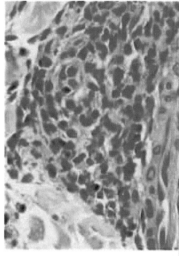

Figure 32c

Adult T-cell leukaemia/lymphoma.
Left-hand panel: Skin immuno-histochemistry (medium power). There is a dense infiltrate of CD3⁺ lymphocytes in the upper dermis. *Right-hand panel:* Skin histopathology (H&E, high power). The lymphocytes display cytological atypia.

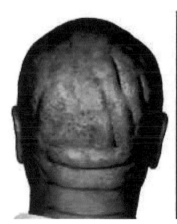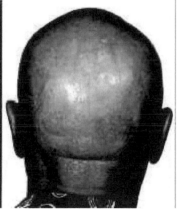

Figure 32d

Erythrodermic adult T-cell leukaemia-lymphoma.
Left: Infiltration of the scalp has produced broad skin folds, an appearance known as cutis verticis gyrata. *Right:* Following treatment with daclizumab, an anti-CD25 antibody, the scalp has returned to normal.

persisted and his general condition deteriorated. Daclizumab (Zenapax), an anti-CD25 antibody, was commenced at a dose of 1 mg/kg, the first 5 doses at weekly intervals and thereafter at monthly intervals. After 3 doses of daclizumab the patient no longer complained of pruritus and both the erythroderma and scaling had resolved (Figure 32d), while a skin biopsy confirmed a histological remission. He remained free from skin lesions and pruritus for 6 months while continuing to receive monthly daclizumab, but suffered a relapse of the skin lesions when the dosing interval was extended to 7 weeks. Although the skin changes responded to a reintroduction of monthly daclizumab administration, the ATLL was never fully controlled and the patient died 18 months after starting biological therapy.

Comment

Adult T-cell leukaemia/lymphoma (ATLL) is a neoplasm of mature T lymphocytes caused by human T-cell leukaemia/lymphoma virus type 1 (HTLV-1) infection, and usually presents with skin lesions, lymphadenopathy and hepatosplenomegaly and with variable involvement of the peripheral blood and bone marrow. HTLV-1 is endemic to parts of Japan, the Southeastern United States, West Africa and the Caribbean basin, where the incidence of ATLL is highest. Transmission of HTLV-1 is via sexual intercourse, blood products, shared needles and breast milk. ATLL develops in 1 per 1000 HTLV-1 carriers per year.

The cutaneous manifestations of ATLL include patches, plaques and tumours as well as an exfoliative erythroderma. The lesions are often indistinguishable from those of HTLV-1-negative cutaneous T-cell lymphomas. Skin histology is heterogenous, including patterns that are similar to mycosis fungoides. The blood film may show the presence of pleiomorphic lymphocytes with multilobulated nuclei, known as 'flower cells'.

Four clinical sub-types of ATLL have been described, referred to as acute, lymphoma-type, chronic and smouldering. Our patient presented with the chronic ATLL; this type, along with the smouldering form, have an indolent course until ultimate progression to acute ATLL. The overall prognosis of ATLL is poor, the mean survival ranging from 6 to 24 months in the acute and chronic forms respectively. Various combinations of cytotoxic chemotherapy have been used to treat ATLL but current regimens offer little overall survival benefit.

Novel treatments for ATLL include monoclonal antibodies, such as dacluzimab, a humanized anti-CD25 antibody. All ATLL cells express CD25, which represents the alpha sub-unit of the interleukin-2 (IL-2) receptor (IL-2Rα). The HTLV-1 *tax* gene indirectly up-regulates transcription of host genes for both IL-2 and IL-2α. Daclizumab may exert its effects by activating antibody-dependent cell-mediated cytotoxicity as well as inhibiting a subset of neoplastic cells whose proliferation depends on autocrine stimulation by IL-2. Although not curative, daclizumab may afford significant symptomatic relief, as in our patient, and appears to possess specific therapeutic activity in the management of ATLL.

Learning points

1. A diagnosis of adult T-cell leukaemia/lymphoma (ATLL) should be considered in an erythrodermic patient from the Caribbean, Japan or West Africa. Clinically the eruption of ATLL may also resemble mycosis fungoides.
2. ATLL is a neoplasm of mature T lymphocytes caused by HTLV-1 infection. Serology can be performed to confirm the presence of HTLV-1 infection while a blood film reveals neoplastic T cells, known as 'flower cells'.
3. ATLL usually progresses to an acute leukaemia, which carries a poor prognosis.

Reference

Setoyama M, Katahira Y, Kanzaki T. Clinicopathologic analysis of 124 cases of adult T-cell leukaemia/lymphoma with cutaneous manifestations. *J Dermatol* 1999; 26: 785–90.

See also case numbers 17, 37, 41.

Case 33

An inflamed toe and a rash on the legs in an immunosuppressed patient

History

A 38-year-old man with chronic myeloid leukaemia received a bone marrow transplant from a matched unrelated donor. On post-transplant day 5 the patient developed acute graft-versus-host-disease, which was treated with high-dose methylprednisolone. On post-transplant day 11 he developed a swollen, red tender left fourth toe with an associated pyrexia. Despite broad-spectrum antibacterial therapy, the toe remained inflamed and became increasingly dusky. On post-transplant day 20 he developed a rash on both legs and a dermatology opinion was requested.

Clinical findings

The skin of the distal and medial aspect of the left fourth toe was gangrenous with grey discoloration extending proximally onto the dorsum of the foot (Figure 33a). There were areas of petechiae and purpura involving both legs (Figures 33b, c). On palpation the lesional skin was associated with multiple subcutaneous, tender nodules. The patient was febrile (38.7°C).

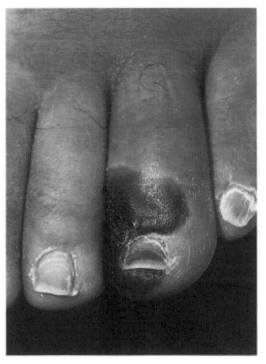

Figure 33a

Fusarium **paronychia.**
This was the primary lesion on the fourth left toe. It commenced as a paronychia, initially erythematous. With time the involved skin became necrotic and was surrounded by a zone of grey discoloration. *Fusarium solani* was cultured from a swab of this skin.

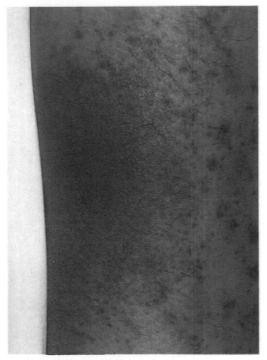

Figure 33b

Disseminated *Fusarium* infection.
A purpuric lesion on the left calf, which
was nodular on palpation. This lesion is
an area of secondary skin infection
following dissemination of *Fusarium*. A
biopsy was sent for histopathology (see
Figure 33d) and culture which grew *F.
solani*.

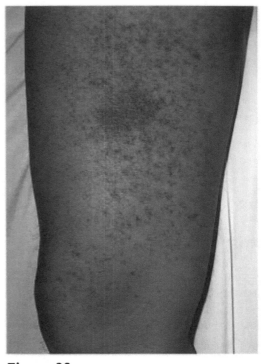

Figure 33c

Disseminated *Fusarium* infection.
Petechiae on the right thigh represent
another area of skin infection
disseminated from the primary fusarial
paronychia.

Investigations

Hb: 9.8 g/dl (11.5–15.5 g/dl), WCC: 3.2×10^9/l
(4.0–11.0×10^9/l), PMN: 0.9×10^9/l (2.5–$7.5 \times$
10^9/l), lymphs: 2.4×10^9/l (1.3–4.0×10^9/l),
plts 33×10^9/l (150–450×10^9/l).

Skin histopathology: Biopsy of a purpuric
lesion on the left calf revealed septate fungal
hyphae in the deep dermis. The fungi demonstrated dichotomous branching (Figure 33d).

Culture of skin biopsy: growth of *Fusarium
solani*.

Swab of left fourth toe: growth of *Fusarium
solani*.

Diagnosis

Disseminated *Fusarium solani* infection.

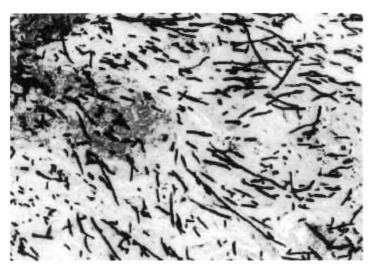

Figure 33d

Disseminated *Fusarium* infection.
Skin histopathology of the purpuric lesion on the left calf (see Figure 33b) (Grocot stain, high power). There are multiple fungal hyphae demonstrating dichotomous branching.

Treatment and progress

The patient was commenced on liposomal amphotericin B and the cutaneous lesions initially improved, but subsequently his clinical condition deteriorated. An abdominal ultrasound demonstrated lesions in his spleen. At laparotomy the spleen was found to contain multiple abscesses, from which *F. solani* was cultured. Thereafter, he developed lung lesions and further skin lesions. Despite continued treatment with liposomal amphotericin B, he died of overwhelming infection 3 months after his transplant.

Comment

Rashes in immunocompromised patients are an important diagnostic problem for the dermatologist. Cutaneous signs may be the harbinger of serious systemic disease and in neutropenic patients bacterial and fungal sepsis must be excluded as a priority.

Fusarium spp. are ubiquitous in nature, occurring in water, the soil and decaying vegetation. They may cause onychomycosis in normal hosts but in the immunocompromised *Fusarium* can become invasive and lead to systemic infection. A number of *Fusarium* spp. have been cultured from tissues of immunosuppressed humans. However, *F. solani* is the most commonly isolated in disseminated disease. Portals of entry include the respiratory tract, via urinary catheters or through skin. The cutaneous route of infection often arises from a *Fusarium* paronychia, as in our case, or from infection of a digital ulcer. At the onset of fusarial skin infection there is an erythematous, inflammatory macule, which, with time, progresses to form an area of dark, necrotic skin or an eschar. The surrounding skin is red or grey. This evolution is a consequence of cutaneous invasion and subsequent thrombosis of dermal vessels by fusarial hyphae. This induces skin necrosis and extravasation of erythrocytes. The tendency to purpura is heightened by thrombocytopenia, which commonly accompanies a generalized reduction in bone marrow function seen in these patients.

In the immunosuppressed about 70% of *Fusarium* infections (including primary skin involvement) will disseminate throughout the body, compared with only about 30% of *Aspergillus* infections. The majority of cases of disseminated *Fusarium* infection occur in patients with haematological malignancies: 85% of patients develop skin lesions, which may take several different forms, including petechiae, violaceous papules, erythematous nodules, keratotic nodules, necrotic ulcers and fluctuant subcutaneous nodules. Skin histology is indistinguishable from that of *Aspergillus* infection, with hyphae demonstrating dichotomous branching and showing a predilection for vascular invasion. Therefore a skin biopsy specimen must be sent for mycological culture.

Fusarium organisms exhibit resistance to many anti-fungal agents and the mortality rate from infection exceeds 70%. The treatment of choice for disseminated *Fusarium* infections is amphotericin B. However, recovery of neutrophil function appears to be the most important factor in resolution. Our patient remained neutropenic throughout his illness despite the use of granulocyte–macrophage colony-stimulating factor.

Learning points

1. Cutaneous lesions are often the earliest manifestations of disseminated fungal infections in immunocompromised patients.
2. A skin biopsy for histopathology provides a rapid diagnosis, whilst tissue sent for culture will yield the pathogenic organism.
3. In the immunocompromised disseminated *Fusarium* infection may follow *Fusarium* paronychia. The skin lesions of *Fusarium* infection are often necrotic or purpuric due to vascular invasion by fungi.

Reference

Bodey GP, Boktour M, Mays S et al. Skin lesions associated with *Fusarium* infection. *Arch Dermatol* 2001; 47: 659–66.

See also case numbers 14, 24.

Case 34
Periorbital erythema following chemotherapy

History

A 30-year-old woman with acute myeloid leukaemia was admitted under the haematologists for the initiation of chemotherapy. Ten days after commencing a regimen of cytarabine, mitoxantrone and etoposide she developed a fever followed by an eruption that started on her left temple and extended to involve the periorbital skin bilaterally. An infectious process was considered the most likely cause and she was given broad spectrum antibiotics and anti-fungal agents. Over the ensuing 48 hours the eruption and fever persisted and so a referral was made to the dermatology department.

Clinical findings

On examination, there were bilateral, symmetrical, erythematous plaques predominantly in a periorbital distribution (Figure 34a). The lesions were well-demarcated, oedematous and tender to touch. The patient had a fever (38.4°C). There was no regional lymphadenopathy.

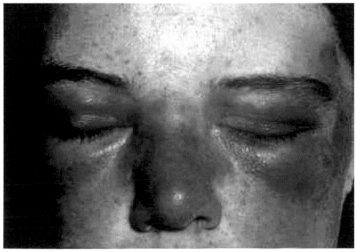

Figure 34a

Neutrophilic eccrine hidradenitis. There is bilateral erythema and swelling around the eyes, which is a characteristic site for this disorder.

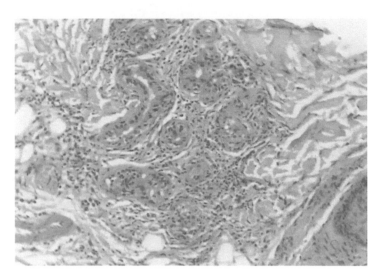

Figure 34b

Neutrophilic eccrine hidradenitis.
Skin histopathology (H&E, medium
power). There is a neutrophil-rich
inflammatory cell infiltrate involving
the secretory coils of an eccrine gland
in the lower dermis.

Investigations

Hb: 10.1 g/dl (11.5–15.5 g/dl), WCC: 1.7 ×
10^9/l (4.0–11.0), PMN: 0.8 × 10^9/l (2.0–7.5 ×
10^9/l), plts: 87 × 10^9/l (150–450 × 10^9/l).

Skin histopathology: A neutrophil-rich
inflammatory cell infiltrate was present
adjacent to the eccrine glands that, at higher
power, was seen to congregate around the
secretory coils destroying the normal glandular architecture. There was cytoplasmic
vacuolation and pyknotic nuclear change in
the basal epidermal cell layer. Periodic acid–
Schiff, Gram and Giemsa stains were
negative (Figure 34b).

Skin biopsy culture: negative.

Blood culture: negative.

Diagnosis

Neutrophilic eccrine hidradenitis.

Treatment and progress

Intravenous methylprednisolone (500 mg
once daily for 3 consecutive days) was given,
which resulted in immediate resolution of
the fever and disappearance of the rash over
the following days. A further course of the
same chemotherapeutic drugs administered
some weeks later was uneventful and did not
produce a reactivation of the rash.

Comment

Neutrophilic eccrine hidradenitis (NEH) is a
characteristic clinicopathological entity
presenting as red plaques and nodules,
usually in a neutropenic patient receiving
chemotherapy for acute myeloid leukaemia.
It occurs typically in the second week
following commencement of chemotherapy
and cytarabine appears to be the most
commonly implicated agent. The eruption

is often accompanied by fever and so must be differentiated from bacterial or fungal sepsis. However, the differential diagnosis includes Sweet's syndrome, pyoderma gangrenosum and leukaemia cutis. Skin histopathology can confirm the diagnosis, demonstrating infiltration of neutrophils around eccrine coils with associated necrosis of the epithelial cells lining the ducts and coils. The condition is often self-limiting and treatment may not be required. However, as in our case, systemic corticosteroids may be prescribed for symptomatic inflammation.

The pathogenesis of drug eruptions based on the eccrine secretory gland remains unclear but is considered to reflect the ability of sweat glands to concentrate chemotherapeutic agents. Drug-induced eccrine cell damage may induce tissue proteases to cleave complement and thus liberate neutrophil chemotactic factors. Eccrine cell necrosis may, in turn, be mediated by release of hydrolytic enzymes from recruited neutrophils. This hypothesis, however, does not explain the localization of NEH to certain sites, mainly the face, neck and upper trunk.

Learning points

1. Neutrophilic eccrine hidradenitis (NEH) occurs as an inflammatory eruption, often involving periorbital skin, in a neutropenic patient receiving chemotherapy (cytarabine) for acute myeloid leukaemia.
2. The diagnosis of NEH is made from a skin biopsy that demonstrates neutrophilic inflammation of the eccrine sweat glands.
3. Despite the presence of fever and neutrophil-rich cutaneous inflammation, bacterial sepsis is absent in NEH and the disorder responds well to systemic corticosteroids.

Reference

Flynn TC, Harrist TJ, Murphy GF et al. Neutrophilic eccrine hidradenitis: a distinctive rash associated with cytarabine therapy and acute leukaemia. *J Am Acad Dermatol* 1984; 11: 584–90.

See also case numbers 8, 17, 20.

Case 35
Nodules and plaques in a boy with progressive liver failure

History

A 9-year-old boy had developed progressive hepatic failure since infancy with obstructive jaundice, hepatosplenomegaly and failure to thrive. The patient's most troubling symptoms were pruritus and the development of numerous, disfiguring cutaneous nodules.

Clinical features

The patient was short and underweight for his age. He displayed dysmorphic, triangular facies, and signs of chronic liver disease, namely, jaundice, palmar erythema and gynaecomastia. Examination of the skin also revealed multiple, pale nodules, most prominent on the face, hands, knees and elbows, where they coalesced to form large plaques (Figures 35a–c).

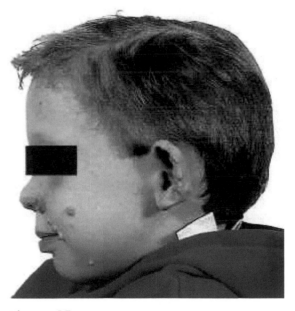

Figure 35a
Alagille syndrome.
There are large nodular xanthomas on the cheeks, nose and ears. Xanthomatosis in AGS arises secondary to cholestastic hyperlipidaemia.

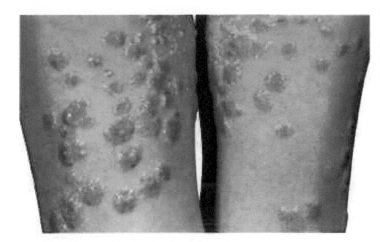

Figure 35b

Alagille syndrome.
On the thighs the xanthomas have
coalesced to form plaques.

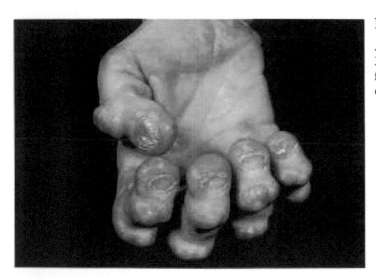

Figure 35c

Alagille syndrome.
Xanthomas over the knuckles cause
functional impairment and
disfigurement.

Investigations

AST: 184 IU/l (10–50 IU/l), GGT: 568 IU/l
(5–55 IU/l), bilirubin: 260 μmol/l (3–20
μmol/l), ALP: 1610 IU/l (30–120 IU/l).

Cholesterol: 19.6 mmol/l (<5.2 mmol/l),
triglycerides: 3.6 mmol/l (<2.3 mmol/l).

Skin histopathology: The epidermis was
normal. There were large aggregates of foam
cells (lipid-rich macrophages) throughout the
dermis. Fibroblasts were increased in
number.

Liver histopathology: There was a generalized paucity of intrahepatic bile ducts.

Diagnosis

Alagille syndrome with xanthomatosis.

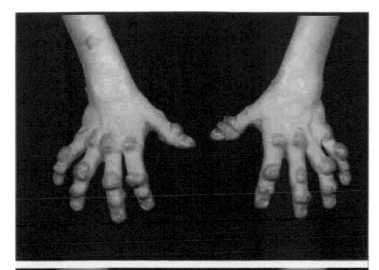

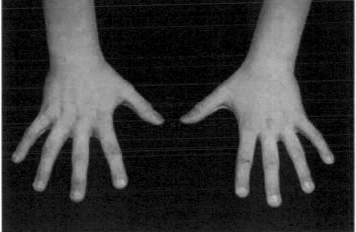

Figure 35d

Alagille syndrome.
Upper panel: Xanthomas on the hands prior to liver transplantation.
Lower panel: Four months post transplant, showing complete clearance of xanthomas.

Treatment and progress

The patient underwent a liver transplant and within hours of the transplant the xanthomas turned dark red and started to shrink. Four months post transplant all had entirely resolved (Figure 35d). Serum cholesterol fell to 3.7 mmol/l within 1 month of the transplant. Palmar erythema, gynaecomastia and pruritus also resolved. Catch-up growth occurred such that at the age of 15 years his height and weight were above the 3rd centile. Ten years after his liver transplant the patient remains well on cyclosporin 80 mg twice daily, azathioprine 25 mg daily and prednisolone 1 mg daily.

Comment

Alagille syndrome (AGS) is an autosomal dominant disorder of biliary hypoplasia leading to cholestatic liver disease. Chronic cholestasis is the principal feature of AGS and results in much of the morbidity of the disease. Intractable pruritus and, as in our case, disfiguring xanthomas markedly reduce the quality of life of children with AGS. Affected individuals also have a number of associated problems, including cardiovascular anomalies (most commonly peripheral pulmonary stenosis), vertebral arch defects, triangular facies, ocular and renal problems. Pruritus and xanthomatosis are generally refractory to medical treatment in AGS and therefore failure to control these symptoms is a major indication for surgical intervention, which includes external biliary diversion as well as liver transplantation.

AGS is caused by mutations in the *Jagged1* (*JAG1*) gene, the disease locus being assigned to 20p12. JAG1 is a cell surface protein that functions as a ligand for the Notch transmembrane receptors. These receptor-ligand pairs are part of the evolutionarily conserved Notch signalling pathway, which functions in many different cell types throughout development to regulate cell fate decisions.

Most children with AGS have facial dysmorphism with a prominent forehead, slight hypertelorism, deeply set eyes, saddle nose and sharp-pointed chin, producing a triangular appearance. The dermatological manifestations of AGS are mostly related to cholestasis or malabsorption. Xanthoma formation is secondary to the hyperlipidaemia: 28% of patients have a serum cholesterol greater than 15 mmol/l and in some it exceeds 40 mmol/l. Hypertriglyceridaemia is less frequent. Coronary heart disease does not appear to be more prevalent despite hyperlipidaemia, due perhaps to the inhibitory effect of ApoE-rich high-density lipoprotein (HDL) particles on platelet aggregation.

Liver transplantation results in an immediate correction of the biochemical abnormality. As in our patient, xanthomas tend to resolve within days to weeks of transplantation. Pruritus also settles rapidly. However, in patients with less severe involvement who do not undergo transplantation, xanthomas have been reported to resolve spontaneously since AGS-associated cholestasis has a tendency to lessen with age.

Learning points

1. Congenital bile duct hypoplasia of Alagille syndrome (AGS) produces severe cholestasis with florid xanthomatosis in early childhood.
2. Patients with AGS possess typical triangular facies with a prominent forehead, hypertelorism and pointed chin.
3. Severe cutaneous complications of AGS (intractable pruritus and disfiguring xanthomatosis) are indications for liver transplant.

Reference

Piccoli DA, Spinner NB. Alagille syndrome and the *Jagged1* gene. *Semin Liver Dis* 2001; 21: 525–8.

See also case numbers 19, 44.

Case 36
A unilateral groin rash

History

An 81-year-old man was referred with a rash involving the right groin. The eruption had been present for a number of years and was mildly pruritic.

Clinical findings

Examination of the right groin demonstrated an extensive erythematous plaque extending from the flexure to the inguinal area. There were areas of crusting on the involved skin. In the centre of the lesion there was a 2 cm diameter erythematous nodule (Figure 36a). There was no regional lymphadenopathy.

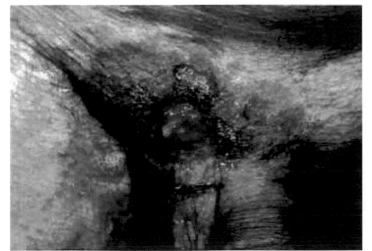

Figure 36a

Extramammary Paget's disease.
There is a 12 cm diameter plaque involving the skin of the right groin and inguinal region bearing a central erythematous nodule and areas of crusting.

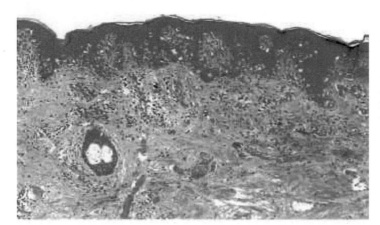

Figure 36b

Extramammary Paget's disease.
Skin histopathology of plaque (H&E, medium power). There is intraepithelial infiltration by small nests of cells and individual malignant Paget cells.

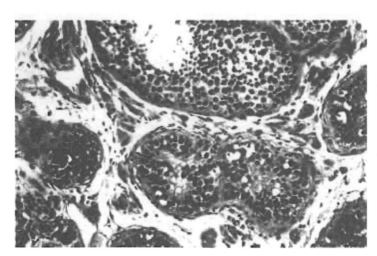

Figure 36c

Extramammary Paget's disease.
Skin histopathology of nodule (H&E, high power). The nodule was an invasive apocrine carcinoma composed of nests of large cells with clear cytoplasm and well-formed glands undergoing luminal secretion.

Investigations

Skin histopathology: Biopsy of the plaque demonstrated a hyperkeratotic and acanthotic epidermis. There was epidermal infiltration by variable numbers of large cells with abundant pale-staining cytoplasm containing large vesicular nuclei (Figure 36b). The cells stained positively with periodic acid–Schiff reaction, indicating the presence of mucopolysaccharides. Biopsy of the nodule demonstrated an invasive adnexal carcinoma showing apocrine differentiation (Figure 36c).

Diagnosis

Extramammary Paget's disease.

Treatment and progress

Colorectal and urogenital examinations were normal with no evidence of internal neoplasia. The lesional skin was excised with a 1 cm margin and the defect corrected by primary closure. At 1 year of follow-up there was no evidence of recurrence.

Comment

Extramammary Paget's disease (EMPD) is a malignant skin condition in which there is intraepidermal infiltration by neoplastic cells showing glandular differentiation. Despite its clinical and histological similarity to Paget's disease of the nipple, EMPD is regarded as a distinct entity. It generally develops in the sixth to ninth decades of life and shows a slight female preponderance. Areas with high density of apocrine glands, namely the vulva, penis, groins, scrotum and perianal skin, are sites of predilection. Clinically, EMPD presents as a unilateral, well-demarcated, scaly and eczematous plaque, which can be several centimetres in diameter. Lesional skin may be exudative and eroded and is often pruritic. EMPD usually progresses slowly over a number of years so that a delay in diagnosis is not uncommon.

Histologically, EMPD is characterized by the presence of intraepithelial neoplastic cells (Paget cells), which possess abundant pale-staining cytoplasm and large atypical nuclei. Paget cells stain positively with PAS, indicating the presence of mucopolysaccharides. Paget cells may be distributed singly or in clusters in the epithelium and there is often extension into hair follicles and sweat gland ducts.

There is a strong relationship between EMPD and adjacent or internal adenocarcinoma. In some patients, as in our case, EMPD occurs in association with an adnexal carcinoma in which Paget cells, derived from an underlying apocrine or eccrine sweat gland tumour, migrate to the epidermis by direct extension. In other cases, EMPD is associated with visceral malignancy in the genitourinary or gastrointestinal tract. However, in this variant there is usually a lack of continuity between EMPD and visceral carcinoma. In the third situation intraepidermal Paget cells occur in the absence of an associated cancer.

The treatment of choice for EMPD is ablative therapy using any one of the following: surgical excision, superficial radiotherapy, curettage, topical 5-fluorouracil, photodynamic therapy, cryosurgery and Moh's micrographic surgery. High rates of local recurrence have been reported following surgery (up to 30% of cases), which reflect the difficulty in delineating clinical margins in EMPD and the multifocal nature of the disease.

Learning points

1. In an elderly patient presenting with a unilateral groin or anogenital dermatosis a biopsy must be performed to exclude a diagnosis of extramammary Paget's disease (EMPD).
2. The diagnosis of EMPD is made by identifying intraepithelial Paget cells on the skin biopsy.
3. EMPD is commonly associated with either a cutaneous adnexal carcinoma or an internal adenocarcinoma of the urogenital or lower gastrointestinal tract. Investigations should be directed at revealing an associated malignancy.

Reference

Balducci L, Crawford EP, Smith GF et al. Extramammary Paget's disease: an annotated review. *Cancer Invest* 1988; 6: 293–303.

See also case number 29.

Case 37
Patches, plaques and lymphadenopathy

History

A 40-year-old man presented with a widespread eruption consisting of scaly patches and plaques scattered over the trunk and limbs (Figure 37a). A biopsy confirmed the clinical diagnosis of mycosis fungoides and over the next few years the dermatosis was successfully managed with intermittent courses of UVB phototherapy and psoralen-UVA (PUVA) photochemotherapy. Ten years after his initial presentation he developed a tender lump in the left groin and over the next few months became unwell with fever, night sweats and weight loss. During this time, his rash improved spontaneously; the red patches faded and the scaling ceased.

Clinical features

On examination, his skin demonstrated widespread mottled and reticulate pigmentation with faint and patchy erythema on the thighs (Figure 37b). He was febrile (37.8°C). There were two large tender lymph nodes in the left inguinal region and hepatomegaly.

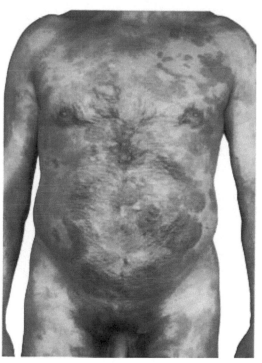

Figure 37a

Mycosis fungoides.
Multiple patches and plaques of mycosis fungoides. The lesions demonstrate typical angulated margins.

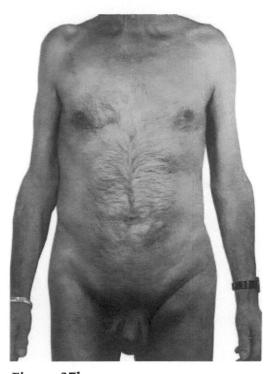

Figure 37b

Hodgkin's disease.
At the time of presentation of the
Hodgkin's disease, the skin lesions of
mycosis fungoides had virtually
disappeared. There is lymphadenopathy in
the left groin.

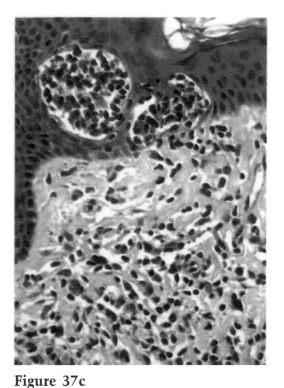

Figure 37c

Mycosis fungoides.
Skin histopathology (H&E, high power).
There are two Pautrier microabscesses
(focal intraepidermal collections of
atypical lymphocytes) in the epidermis
and a dermal infiltrate of abnormal
lymphocytes, consistent with mycosis
fungoides.

Investigations

Hb: 8.7 g/dl (11.5–15.5 g/dl), WCC: 6.8×10^9/l
(4.0–11.0 $\times 10^9$/l), plts: 735×10^9/l (150–450
$\times 10^9$/l), ESR: 134 mm/hr (1–10 mm/hr).

Ultrasound abdomen: hepatomegaly.

Skin histopathology: Biopsy of a patch
demonstrated a dermal infiltrate of atypical
lymphocytes displaying epidermotropism
and focal intraepidermal aggregation
(Pautrier microabscesses) (Figure 37c).

Lymph node histopathology: Biopsy of a
groin node showed a dense infiltrate of reticulum
cells, lymphoid cells and eosinophils
together with numerous Reed–Sternberg
cells (Figure 37d).

Diagnosis

1. **Mycosis fungoides (skin).**
2. **Mixed cellularity Hodgkin's disease
   (lymph node).**

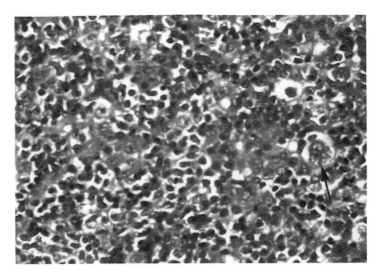

Figure 37d

Hodgkin's disease.
Lymph node histopathology (H&E, high power). There are numerous Reed–Sternberg cells (arrow) with a scattered population of mixed inflammatory cells, consistent with mixed cellularity Hodgkin's disease.

Treatment and progress

The patient received combination chemotherapy for the Hodgkin's disease with chlorambucil, vincristine, procarbazine and prednisolone with a good clinical response and clearance of the skin lesions. Two years later the Hodgkin's disease was still in remission but the mycosis fungoides (MF) had relapsed and had necessitated the use of further PUVA. Over the next 10 years of follow-up there was no relapse of the Hodgkin's disease; however, the patient continued to receive treatment for the MF.

Comment

Mycosis fungoides (MF) is the most common of the cutaneous T-cell lymphomas. Usually, the disease is limited to the skin alone and persists for many years, often indefinitely. Dissemination to lymph nodes, liver and spleen occurs in advanced stages, usually in the context of extensive cutaneous involvement with widespread plaques, tumours or erythroderma. Hodgkin's disease (HD) is a lymphoid neoplasm, arising in lymph nodes, composed of mononuclear Hodgkin cells and multinucleated Reed–Sternberg cells. In more than 98% of Hodgkin's lymphomas the neoplastic cells are derived from mature B cells at the germinal centre stage of differentiation. In rare cases they are derived from peripheral T cells. Cutaneous HD is infrequent and typically occurs in skin drained by lymph nodes already extensively involved by HD. In our case lymphadenopathy developed in a patient with a pre-existing cutaneous T-cell lymphoma. However, lymph node analysis revealed the presence of a second, systemic Hodgkin's lymphoma.

The association between MF and HD was first reported in 1963 and since then numerous cases have been reported. As in our case, mycosis fungoides lesions usually appear before those of Hodgkin's disease, but the reverse has also been documented. The association between these two forms of lymphoma has led to speculation that MF and HD are derived from the same clone. Investigation of two cases similar to our own has demonstrated divergent immunophenotypes and gene rearrangements indicating that the lymphomas are not derived from a common clone.

A remarkable feature of our case was the clinical regression of the mycosis fungoides as the Hodgkin's disease developed. There is no clear explanation for this phenomenon. However, functional T-cell defects are well documented in HD and could perhaps account for the regression of our patient's MF. An inverse relationship between the two lymphomas is further illustrated by a recrudescence of the MF once the HD was in remission.

Learning points

1. A lymph node biopsy is mandatory in a patient with mycosis fungoides (MF) who develops lymphadenopathy.
2. Second lymphomas, such as Hodgkin's disease, may occur concurrently with MF.
3. The long-term prognosis of MF is generally good.

Reference

Brousset P, Lamant L, Viraben R et al. Hodgkin's disease following mycosis fungoides: phenotypic and molecular evidence for different tumour cell clones. *J Clin Pathol* 1996; 49: 504–7.

See also case numbers 32, 41.

Case 38
A plaque on the shin

History

A 67-year-old woman, otherwise in good health, presented with a tender plaque on her left shin that had been gradually enlarging for the past 18 months. She had noticed a susceptibility to bruising within the lesion following minimal trauma.

Clinical findings

Examination revealed a 4 cm diameter yellow-brown plaque on the left shin that had a waxy, rather gelatinous appearance, but was firm and indurated on palpation (Figures 38a, b). Purpura was readily produced within the lesion. The rest of the skin examination was normal.

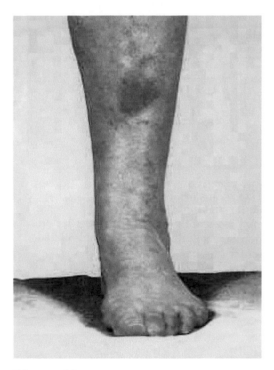

Figure 38a

Nodular amyloid.
There is a yellow–brown plaque on the left shin.

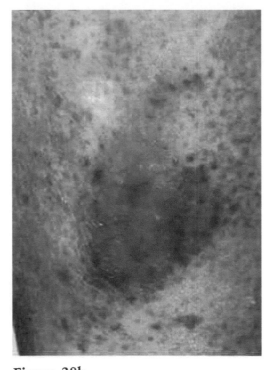

Figure 38b

Nodular amyloid.
Ecchymoses are present within the lesion,
which is a telltale sign of amyloid-related
vascular fragility.

Investigations

Skin histopathology: Large masses of
amorphous eosinophilic material were
identified throughout the entire dermis.
When stained with Congo red and viewed
under polarized light, apple-green birefringence was seen, confirming the presence of
amyloid (Figure 38c). A chronic inflammatory cell infiltrate consisting mostly of
plasma cells was present within lesional
dermis.

FBC: normal, U&E: normal, LFT: normal.
ESR: normal.

Serum immunoglobulins: normal.

Serum protein electrophoresis: normal.

Urinary Bence-Jones protein analysis:
negative.

Bone marrow biopsy: normal.

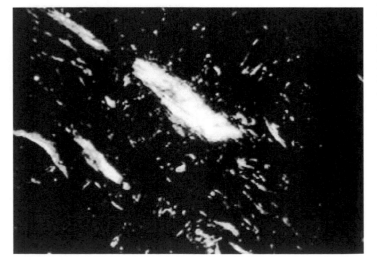

Figure 38c

Nodular amyloid.
Skin histopathology (Congo red, high
power). Examination of the dermal
material under polarized light reveals
apple-green birefringence confirming
amyloid.

Diagnosis

Nodular amyloid.

Treatment and progress

In view of the site and size of the lesion, no treatment was undertaken. The patient was recommended to use a footballer's shin pad to protect the lesion. Regular follow-up over several years did not demonstrate further expansion of the lesion or the development of a systemic plasma cell dyscrasia.

Comment

Primary cutaneous amyloidosis consists of three types: nodular, macular and lichenoid, of which the nodular (or tumefactive) form is the rarest. Nodular amyloidosis can present as either a solitary lesion, as in our case, or as multiple nodules or plaques. Lesions can occur at any site but are typically found on the legs, face and trunk. The lesions are yellow–brown or pink, waxy in appearance and firm on palpation, and frequently have surface telangiectasiae. The disorder most commonly develops during the sixth and seventh decades and women are affected twice as often as men. Nodular amyloid is quite distinct from the other forms of primary cutaneous amyloid: macular amyloid is typified by rippled macular hyperpigmentation, whilst lichen amyloid presents as an eruption of monomorphic lichenoid papules. Histologically, amyloid deposition in the nodular form is present throughout the entire dermis – again in contrast to the other primary cutaneous amyloidoses, where only superficial dermal involvement is seen.

Immunohistochemical studies have demonstrated that the amyloid fibrils in nodular amyloid are derived from immunoglobulin light chains and are consequently of protein AL (light chain amyloid) type as found in primary and myeloma-associated systemic amyloidosis. It has therefore been suggested that nodular amyloid could be regarded as an extramedullary plasmacytoma in which amyloid fibrils are produced locally by plasma cells. In other cases the nodular amyloid fibril protein has been characterized as polyclonal, suggesting that the nodular deposit is secondary to reactive rather than neoplastic plasma cell expansion.

There is an infrequent progression of nodular lesions to systemic amyloidosis, and it has therefore been proposed that patients should be kept under regular follow-up and investigated with regular immunoglobulin evaluation and intermittent bone marrow analysis.

In view of the localized nature of nodular amyloid, lesions can be removed surgically via excision or curettage; however, recurrence is not uncommon.

Learning points

1. Provocation of purpura with minimal trauma should raise the suspicion of cutaneous amyloid.
2. Nodular amyloid is the rarest form of primary cutaneous amyloidosis, the other types being macular and lichenoid.
3. Nodular amyloid may progress to a systemic plasma cell dyscrasia; therefore patients need to be kept under regular, long-term follow-up.

Reference

Touart DM, Sau P. Cutaneous deposition diseases. *J Am Acad Dermatol* 1998; 39: 149–59.

See also case number 4.

Case 39
A rash and numbness involving the right thumb

History

A 31-year-old Indian woman developed numbness of the lateral border of the right thumb three weeks after a full-term delivery. The pregnancy had been uncomplicated and her baby was healthy. Following the onset of sensory symptoms, an erythematous, papular eruption appeared on the skin of the thumb. She went on to complain of further localized symptoms, including swelling of the right wrist, loss of right-hand grip strength and loss of sensation in the right thumb.

Clinical findings

There were groups of confluent, smooth papules forming flat, red–brown plaques over the medial and dorsal aspects of the right thumb (Figure 39a). Further papules were scattered around the base of the thumb. Neurological examination revealed an absence of light touch, pinprick and temperature sensation over the lateral border of the thumb. The right radial cutaneous and right median nerves were thickened and tender. Tinel's sign of the right median nerve (the induction of sharp pain by tapping a nerve) was positive at the wrist. Power was significantly reduced in the right abductor pollicis brevis muscle.

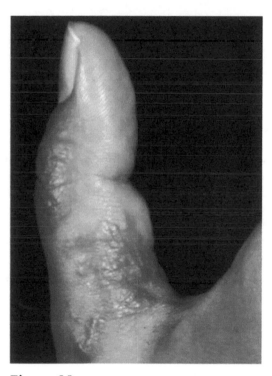

Figure 39a

Borderline tuberculoid leprosy.
There are well-defined, smooth, red–brown plaques on the medial and dorsal surfaces of the right thumb. Sensation over the thumb was diminished.

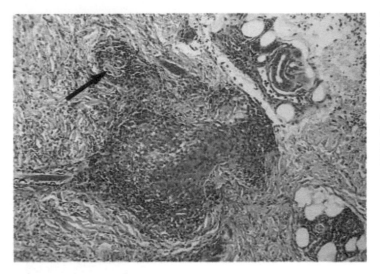

Figure 39b

Borderline tuberculoid leprosy.
(H&E, high power). There is a loose, non-caseating granuloma of epithelioid cells in the deep dermis. There is an infiltrate of inflammatory cells surrounding and invading a nearby nerve twig (arrowed). Stains for mycobacteria (Wade–Fite, Zeihl–Neilson) were negative.

Investigations

Skin histopathology: Biopsy of the plaque revealed confluent oedematous granulomas through the mid dermis with sparing of the papillary dermis. There was evidence of neurotropism and nerve destruction. No mycobacteria were seen with special stains (Wade–Fite, Zeihl–Neilson) (Figure 39b).

Nerve conduction studies demonstrated median nerve damage.

Diagnosis

Borderline tuberculoid leprosy in reaction.

Treatment and progress

The patient was treated with the World Health Organization recommended regimen for paucibacillary leprosy: rifampicin 600 mg monthly together with dapsone 100 mg daily.

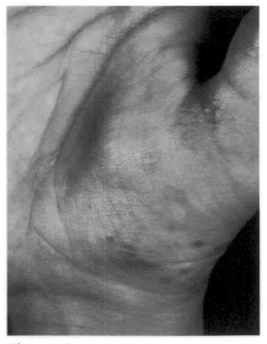

Figure 39c

Borderline tuberculoid leprosy.
There is a 2 cm diameter swelling over the right thenar eminence. This was a nerve abscess involving the median nerve. It subsequently discharged spontaneously. There are satellite skin lesions at the base of the thumb and at the wrist.

She was commenced on prednisolone 40 mg daily for the management of the neuritis; however, this had to be discontinued due to upper gastrointestinal side-effects. She subsequently developed a tender 2 cm fixed nodule over the right thenar eminence (Figure 39c). Magnetic resonance imaging (MRI) of the hand demonstrated thickening of the median nerve with an associated nerve abscess at the site of the nodule (Figure 39d). She was restarted on oral prednisolone and subsequently the nerve abscess discharged. Over the ensuing months her skin lesions settled and the median nerve function improved.

Comment

The spectrum of signs and symptoms seen in leprosy reflects the wide variation in patients' ability to mount an immune response to *Mycobacterium leprae.* In tuberculoid forms the host delivers a cellular response with a Th1 cytokine profile that induces relative protection against mycobacteria. Histologically, there is a granulomatous infiltrate and an absence of lepromatous bacilli. In borderline tuberculoid disease immunological resistance is strong enough to restrain the infection but is insufficient to induce complete clearance. This form of leprosy is unstable and tends to enter a reactional state, either upgrading to tuberculoid disease or downgrading to a borderline lepromatous form. The type I (lepra) reaction, as seen in our patient, is characterized by increased erythema of skin lesions, the onset of neuritis and, sometimes, constitutional symptoms. Type I reactions are encountered in certain circumstances, such as pregnancy and following initiation of effective anti-lepromatous therapy. Our patient presented shortly after delivery with the development of localized sensory symptoms, inflammatory papules and finally a tender, swollen wrist, the latter being a manifestation of

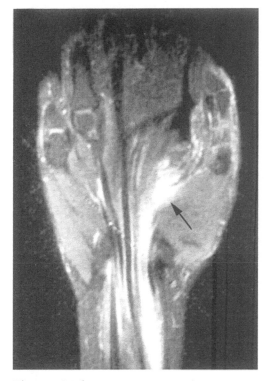

Figure 39d

Borderline tuberculoid leprosy.
Magnetic resonance imaging (MRI) of the right hand and wrist demonstrates enhancement and thickening of the median nerve. The abscess is revealed as a focus of high signal intensity adjacent to the thenar musculature (*arrow*).

median nerve neuritis. In pregnancy there is relative immunosuppression, with the maternal immune response being directed away from cell-mediated immunity to humoral activity. With restoration of full cell-mediated immunity in the immediate post-partum period, sub-clinical symptoms become manifest. Recognition of covert antigen within peripheral nerves results in neuritis and nerve damage. Nerve abscess formation is unusual and appears to be due to an exacerbation of an existing lepromatous lesion or secondary to necrosis in a neural granuloma.

The cutaneous lesions of borderline tuberculoid (BT) leprosy typically consist of plaques and papules. As in tuberculoid (TT) disease, the borders of plaques in BT leprosy are sharply delineated, but, in contrast to TT, satellite papules occur, as in our case. Furthermore, BT lesions tend to be less scaly, red, indurated and raised than TT lesions. Loss of sensation in skin lesions is the rule and regional nerve involvement with enlargement and palsies is common.

Reference

Lockwood DNJ, Sinha HH. Pregnancy and leprosy: a comprehensive literature review. *Int J Lepr* 1999; 67: 6–12.

See also case number 11.

Learning points

1. In tuberculoid forms of leprosy, resistance to *M. leprae* is high, small numbers of organisms are present and skin lesions are few. Histopathology of a skin biopsy reveals granulomatous inflammation, often showing neurotropism.
2. Pregnancy is a recognized precipitating factor for leprosy due to a relatively reduced immunity. In the post-partum period type I reactions (characterized by sudden enhanced inflammation of skin lesions and neuritis) can occur when normal immune function is restored.
3. In borderline tuberculoid leprosy satellite papules are often found adjacent to the main plaques.

Case 40

Widespread skin sloughing in a man with fits

History

A 34-year-old man from the Ivory Coast was admitted with a 1-day history of grand mal seizures. The previous day he had suffered a severe headache. A CT scan of the brain demonstrated an enhancing ring lesion in the right parietal lobe. A diagnosis of cerebral toxoplasmosis was suspected and the patient was commenced on intravenous sulpha-diazine and pyrimethine. Phenytoin was introduced to control the seizures. Three days later he developed a fever, a sore mouth and red eyes. Over the following days the patient developed a widespread, itchy skin eruption.

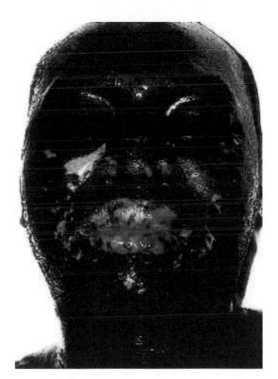

Figure 40a

Toxic epidermal necrolysis.
Involvement of the lips is prominent in TEN. In this African patient the denuded, pink dermis is visible on the lips and right cheek.

Clinical findings

The patient was ill with a high fever (38.8°C). Examination revealed severe haemorrhagic mucositis of the mouth and lips and injection of the conjunctivae (Figure 40a). There were extensive areas of dusky erythema on his trunk and face and large, flaccid blisters on the arms and legs (Figures 40b). The dermatosis involved approximately 40% of the total body surface area.

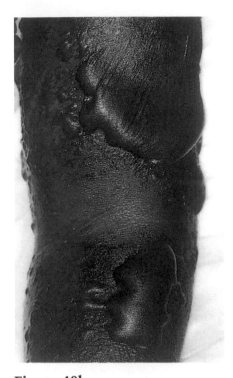

Figure 40b

Toxic epidermal necrolysis.
Large flaccid bullae, such as these on the left arm, developed extensively on the limbs.

Investigations

Hb: 9.5 g/dl (11.5–15.5 g/dl), WCC: 4.1 × 10^9/l (4.0–11.0 × 10^9/l), lymphs: 0.45 × 10^9/1.3–4.0 × 10^9/l, plts: 286 × 10^9/l (150–450 × 10^9/l). ESR: 54 mm/hr (1–10 mm/hr).

Serum creatinine: 136 μmol/l (40–120 μmol/l).

Albumin: 27 g/l (35–50 g/l), GGT: 601 IU/l (5–55 IU/l), AST: 169 IU/l (10–50 IU/l).

CT brain scan: a solitary enhancing ring lesion was present in the right parietal lobe (Figure 40d).

Toxoplasmosis IgG: positive.

HIV-1 serology: positive.

Skin histopathology: There was a subepidermal bulla with overlying confluent necrosis of the epidermis and a sparse perivascular infiltrate of lymphocytes (Figure 40e).

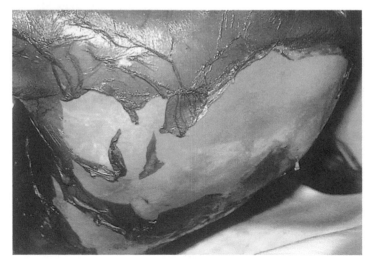

Figure 40c

Toxic epidermal necrolysis
Progressive epidermal necrolysis resulted in complete denudation of the back revealing exposed dermis. Involvement of a large surface area in TEN results in a significant loss of fluid, protein and heat. (This image is from another TEN patient with a similar degree of involvement; *courtesy of the St John's Institute of Dermatology.*)

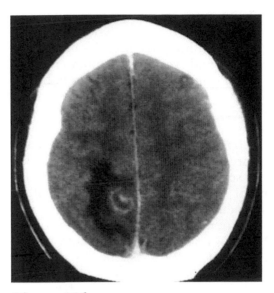

Figure 40d

Cerebral toxoplasmosis.
CT scan brain. This patient presented
with fits secondary to cerebral
toxoplasmosis, which is seen in this image
as a ring lesion with surrounding oedema
in the right parietal lobe. He was
subsequently found to be HIV-positive.
TEN developed following treatment with
sulphadiazine and phenytoin.

Diagnosis

Toxic epidermal necrolysis.

Treatment and progress

Two drugs were implicated in this adverse
reaction: phenytoin and sulphadiazine. Both
were stopped immediately and substituted
by sodium valproate and clindamycin respectively.

The patient was barrier-nursed on a
pressure-relieving mattress. Regular record-
ings of blood pressure and urine output
guided intravenous fluid replacement. He
also received nasogastric feeding. Opiate
analgesia was administered for skin pain. A
greasy emollient (50:50 white soft paraffin/
liquid paraffin) was applied frequently to the
total skin surface. Twice a day the skin was
bathed in 0.05% chlorhexidine solution. The
mouth was toileted frequently and benzy-
damine hydrochloride spray was used hourly

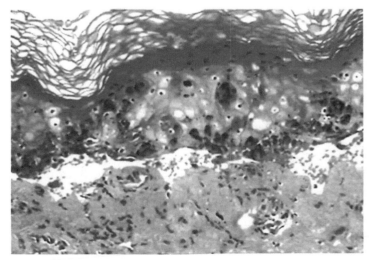

Figure 40e

Toxic epidermal necrolysis.
Skin histopathology (H&E, medium
power). There is a sub-epidermal
blister containing erythrocytes. The
epidermis shows full-thickness
necrosis. The underlying dermis
contains a modest lymphocytic
infiltrate.

to relieve buccal pain. To the eyes dexamethasone drops were applied 6-hourly and chloramphenical ointment 12-hourly. In an attempt to limit the epidermal sloughing, intravenous immunoglobulin was given at a dose of 2 g/kg over 2 days.

Despite active treatment, the total area of blistering and epidermal denudation increased to 50–60% body surface area (Figure 40c). Denuded areas were covered with a silicone mesh dressing. On day 6 of the illness, the patient became hypotensive (blood pressure: 90/45). A skin swab and a blood culture grew *Klebsiella* spp. This responded to ticarcillin.

Eight days after the diagnosis was made there was evidence of re-epithelialization, which was complete 1 week later. The patient recovered well with resolution of renal and hepatic function. He was commenced on anti-retroviral therapy.

Comment

Toxic epidermal necrolysis (TEN) is a life-threatening drug hypersensitivity syndrome characterized by blistering and confluent epidermal sloughing of greater than 30% body surface area. TEN is associated with considerable morbidity and a mortality rate of approximately 25% (mostly from sepsis or multi-organ failure). TEN appears to have a higher incidence in patients with HIV-1 infection, particularly in those treated with sulphonamides, anti-convulsants and certain anti-retroviral agents, such as nevirapine. Clustering of cases of TEN in HIV reflects both an exaggerated sensitivity to drugs among these patients and an increased prescription of high-risk medicines.

Clinically, the initial symptoms of TEN include fever, conjunctivitis, sore throat and widespread itching. Thereafter, clinically evident epithelial necrosis ensues, with the mucous membranes being involved first.

Skin involvement generally begins on the face, upper trunk or acral regions and is characterized by dusky red macules or target-like lesions. Small vesicles are often present in the initial stages and may progress to large flaccid bullae. Over the next few days there is widespread epidermal detachment leaving large areas of exposed and exudative dermis. Re-epithelialization takes place over 14 days, with skin involvement tending to heal without scar formation whereas mucosal scarring of the eyes can lead to potentially disabling ocular sequelae.

The loss of an extensive area of epidermis in TEN is associated with 'acute skin failure', a term used to describe the visceral manifestations that result from widespread epithelial denudation. Release of inflammatory mediators induces high fever while 'stress' hormones increase catabolism and may lead to insulin resistance with hyperglycaemia. Impairment of the barrier function results in impaired thermoregulation and loss of water and electrolytes (50% epidermal detachment results in approximately 2–3 litres of evaporative water loss per day). The exposed dermis may become colonized by bacteria, which, if untreated, can penetrate the vasculature and result in serious systemic sepsis. Epithelial necrosis in other sites can result in gastrointestinal and bronchial mucosal sloughing. Other systemic complications include anaemia, acute renal failure, hepatitis, acute pancreatitis and thromboembolism.

Many drugs have been implicated in the pathogenesis of TEN. However, the most common culprits are sulphonamides, anti-convulsant agents, allopurinol and oxicam non-steroidal anti-inflammatory drugs. Our patient received sulphadiazine to treat cerebral toxoplasmosis and phenytoin to suppress the associated epilepsy. Both drugs could be implicated and so both were discontinued. Studies have demonstrated that early cessation of the offending drug can significantly reduce the extent of TEN.

Epidermal necrosis in TEN results from keratinocyte apoptosis mediated by interactions between the cell membrane death receptor Fas and its ligand, FasL. Normal human immunoglobulin inhibits keratinocyte apoptosis by blocking the Fas receptor. Therapeutic trials have suggested that intravenous immunoglobulin treatment, if given early in the disease, may modify epidermal necrolysis and improve outcome. However, despite therapeutic advances, intensive supportive care remains the main principle of management in TEN.

Reference

Garcia-Doval I, LeCleach L, Bocquet H et al. Toxic epidermal necrolysis and Stevens–Johnson syndrome. *Arch Dermatol* 2000; 136: 232–237.

See also case numbers 42, 47.

Learning points

1. Toxic epidermal necrolysis (TEN) is the most severe cutaneous adverse drug reaction. Early recognition and immediate withdrawal of the suspected drug(s) will limit the extent of involvement.
2. Patients infected with HIV-1 have a higher risk of developing TEN.
3. Principles of therapy include fluid replacement, nutritional support, skin care and treatment of superadded infection. Intravenous immunoglobulin may modify epidermal necrolysis by inhibiting keratinocyte apoptosis.

Case 41
A plaque on the chest

History

A 65-year-old man presented with a 5-month history of an enlarging, itchy lesion on his left upper chest. He reported that, although growing, there were areas within the lesion that were spontaneously healing. Just prior to presentation two smaller, similar lesions had developed close by the original plaque. He was otherwise well.

Clinical findings

On the skin overlying the left pectoral region there was a 5 cm diameter horseshoe-shaped plaque (Figure 41a). The lesional tissue was indurated and red with surface telangiectasiae. Within the lesion were signs of spontaneous clearing. There were two satellite nodules beneath the larger plaque. There was no regional lymphadenopathy.

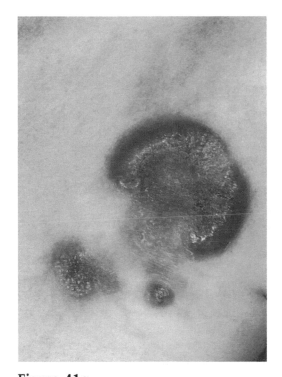

Figure 41a

Primary cutaneous anaplastic large cell lymphoma.
The patient initially presented with an erythematous, indurated horseshoe-shaped plaque on the chest. There had been spontaneous clearing within the lesion.

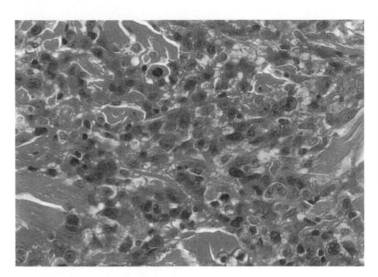

Figure 41b

Primary cutaneous anaplastic large cell lymphoma.
Skin histopathology (H&E, high power). Within the dermis and subcutis is a dense infiltrate of large anaplastic lymphoid cells dissecting the collagen bundles. Mononuclear and binuclear tumour cells are present which show multiple atypical mitoses.

Investigations

Hb: 11.8 g/dl (11.5–15.5 g/dl), WCC: 6.2 × 10⁹/l (4.0–11.0 × 10⁹/l), plts: 366 × 10⁹/l (150–450 × 10⁹/l). ESR: 37 mm/hr (1–10 mm/hr).

Chest x-ray: normal.

CT chest, abdomen, pelvis: normal.

Skin histopathology: Throughout the dermis and subcutis there was a dense infiltrate of large lymphoid cells with highly pleomorphic vesicular nuclei displaying multiple, atypical mitoses (Figure 41b). The infiltrate did not demonstrate epidermotropism. Immunohistochemical analysis revealed the tumour cells to be positive for CD30 but negative for anaplastic lymphoma kinase-1 (ALK1) and epithelial membrane antigen (EMA) (Figure 41c).

Treatment and progress

The patient initially failed to attend for treatment. However, ultimately he was persuaded to accept therapy, but by this time, which was 4 months following presentation, the lesions had enlarged and become tumid (Figure 41d). There was also regional lymphadenopathy. Histopathology of a lymph node demonstrated an infiltrate similar to the skin pathology with large pleomorphic cells staining positively for CD30. He received 6 cycles of CHOP chemotherapy (cyclophosphamide, doxorubicin, vincristine and prednisone) which produced a dramatic reduction in the size of the cutaneous lesions and complete resolution of the lymphadenopathy. A residual cutaneous nodule was cleared with superficial radiotherapy. There has been no evidence of relapse after 3 years of follow-up.

Diagnosis

Primary cutaneous anaplastic large cell lymphoma.

Comment

Primary cutaneous anaplastic large cell lymphoma (ALCL) is a T-cell neoplasm

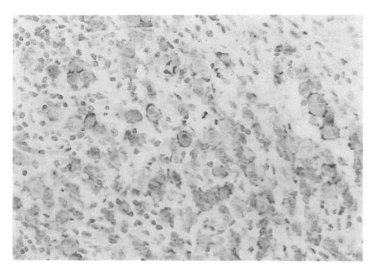

Figure 41c

Primary cutaneous anaplastic large cell lymphoma.
Skin immunohistochemistry (high power). The tumour cells show a strong positive reaction for CD30. The tumour cells were negative for ALK1 and EMA. This pattern of immunoreactivity supports a diagnosis of primary cutaneous anaplastic large cell lymphoma.

consisting of CD30⁺ lymphoid cells. Clinically, primary cutaneous ALCL presents with solitary or localized skin lesions, as in our case, which may be nodular or tumid. The condition usually has an indolent course with an overall 5-year survival rate of 90%. Extracutaneous dissemination occurs in approximately 10% of cases and is an unfavourable prognostic indicator. Approximately 25% of patients will show partial or complete spontaneous regression, but this may be followed by subsequent relapse.

At presentation, it is important to distinguish primary cutaneous ALCL from systemic ALCL with cutaneous involvement by appropriate staging investigations, including CT imaging, lymph node biopsy, bone marrow sampling and immunohistochemistry of lesional tissue. In systemic ALCL tumour cells are positive for ALK1 (the gene product of the pathogenetic t(2;5) translocation) whereas in primary cutaneous ALCL tumour cells are negative for ALK1. In addition, most primary cutaneous cases are negative for EMA whereas systemic ALCL is usually positive for EMA.

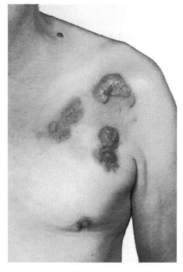

Figure 41d

Primary cutaneous anaplastic large cell lymphoma.
There was a gap of 4 months between presentation (Figure 41a) and initiation of treatment. During this time the lesions expanded and became tumid. Lymph nodes were palpable in the left axilla and left supraclavicular fossa. A lymph node biopsy demonstrated the presence of CD30⁺ anaplastic lymphoma.

Lymphomatoid papulosis (LyP), another primary cutaneous CD30⁺ lymphoproliferative disorder, is a chronic, recurrent, self-healing papulonodular dermatosis that relapses and remits over a long period. Between 10% and 20% of LyP cases will be complicated by the development of a lymphoma. In some cases lesions may become tumid and be histologically indistinguishable from primary cutaneous ALCL, the so-called 'LyP type C'. Since the clinical, histological and immunohistochemical features of primary cutaneous ALCL and LyP can overlap, these conditions may represent a spectrum of primary cutaneous CD30⁺ lymphoproliferative diseases.

In the management of primary cutaneous ALCL with limited disease, skin-directed therapies are recommended, such as radiotherapy or surgical excision. Multi-agent chemotherapy should be reserved for cases with extracutaneous involvement.

Learning points

1. Primary cutaneous anaplastic large cell lymphoma (ALCL) presents as a solitary tumour or a localized collection of nodules. This lymphoma has a tendency to self-resolution and, generally, a good prognosis.
2. The diagnosis of primary cutaneous ALCL is based on histological and immunohistochemical analysis of a skin biopsy. Typically the tumour cells are positive for CD30 but negative for ALK1 and EMA.
3. Primary cutaneous CD30⁺ lymphoproliferative disorders probably constitute a spectrum with primary cutaneous ALCL at one end and lymphomatoid papulosis at the other.

Reference

Bekkenk MW, Geelen FAMJ, van Voorst Vader PC et al. Primary and secondary cutaneous CD30⁺ lymphoproliferative disorders. *Blood* 2000; 95: 3653–61.

See also case numbers 17, 32, 37.

Case 42
A polymorphic mucocutaneous eruption in a patient with lymphoma

History

A 65-year-old man presented with a 3-week history of a widespread eruption involving the skin of the face, trunk and limbs. The patient had also developed soreness of his mouth, bleeding of the lips, dry eyes and visual disturbance. Two years earlier he had been diagnosed with a lymphoplasmacytic lymphoma and Waldenström's macroglobulinaemia, for which he received chlorambucil and regular plasmapheresis.

Clinical findings

Examination revealed superficial erosions on the face (Figure 42a) and discrete blisters on his forearms. There was a widespread lichenoid eruption on the torso with eroded areas on the upper chest and proximal arms (Figure 42b). Palmo–plantar skin was involved with hyperkeratosis and desquamation (Figure 42c). Examination of the eyes revealed injection of the conjunctivae and erosions of the eyelid margins. There was diffuse inflammation of the tongue, erosions on the palatal mucous membranes and haemorrhagic crusting of the lips (Figure 42d).

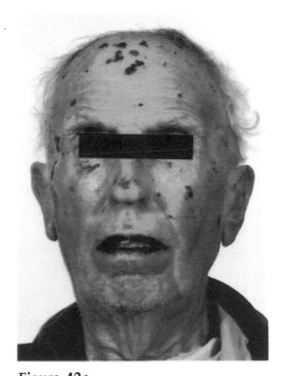

Figure 42a

Paraneoplastic pemphigus.
On presentation, the patient was noted to have erosions of his scalp and cheeks and haemorrhagic mucositis of his lips.

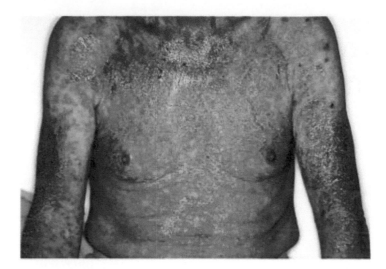

Figure 42b

Paraneoplastic pemphigus.
On presentation, there was a widespread lichenoid eruption on the trunk and limbs of this patient with an underlying lymphoplasmacytic lymphoma.

Investigations

Hb: 9.6 g/dl (11.5–15.5 g/dl), WCC: 3.6 × 10⁹/l (4.0–11.0 × 10⁹/l), PMN: 3.3 × 10⁹/l (2.0–7.5 × 10⁹/l), lymphs: 0.3 × 10⁹/l (1.3–4.0 × 10⁹/l), plts: 24 × 10⁹/l (150–450 × 10⁹/l). ESR: 74 mm/hr (1–10 mm/hr)

IgM: 6.8 g/l (0.49–2.0 g/l), IgA, IgG: reduced.

Autoantibodies: negative.

ENA: negative.

CT scan of thorax, abdomen and pelvis: Extensive and bulky para-aortic and inguinal lymphadenopathy

Histopathology of skin: Biopsy through the margin of a blister showed sub-epidermal blistering with intraepidermal acantholysis. Biopsy through the lichenoid eruption showed a lymphocytic interface inflammatory reaction with associated basal vacuolar degeneration.

Histopathology of oral mucosa: There was intraepithelial blistering with acantholysis (Figure 42e).

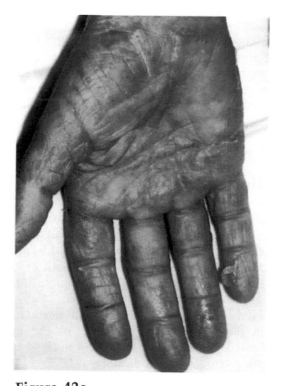

Figure 42c

Paraneoplastic pemphigus.
Acral involvement is prominent with inflammation of palmar skin producing desquamation.

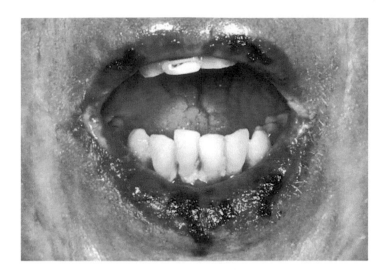

Figure 42d

Paraneoplastic pemphigus.
Haemorrhagic crusting of the lips reflects mucous membrane involvement.

Direct immunofluorescence of skin: This showed intercellular and basement membrane zone deposition of IgG and complement (C3) (Figure 42f).

Indirect immunofluorescence: This showed binding of circulating autoantibodies to normal human skin, rat bladder and monkey oesophagus.

Immunoblotting: This identified 250, 230, 210 and 190 kDa proteins in the patient's serum.

Diagnosis

Paraneoplastic pemphigus.

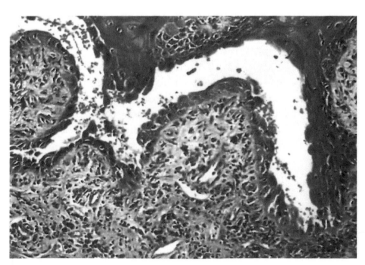

Figure 42e

Paraneoplastic pemphigus.
Oral mucous membrane histopathology (H&E, medium power). There is an intraepithelial cleft with dermal papillae simulating 'villi' as they protrude into the cleft. The keratinocytes show acantholysis.

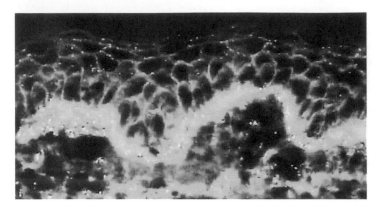

Figure 42f

Paraneoplastic pemphigus.
Direct immunofluorescence: There is intercellular and basement membrane zone deposition of IgG. There was a similar pattern of C3 immunoreactivity.

Treatment and progress

Systemic therapy was instituted with mycophenolate mofetil 500 mg twice daily and intravenous immunoglobulin administered at a dose of 2 g/kg given over 2 days. Topical therapy consisted of frequent use of a greasy emollient and twice-daily applications of a superpotent topical corticosteroid. Corticosteroid eyedrops and mouthwashes were also used twice daily. There was some initial improvement on combined systemic and topical therapy with, in particular, clearance of the lichenoid eruption. However, after 1 week of therapy new blisters appeared and so the patient underwent plasmapheresis and received pulsed methylprednisolone 500 mg on 3 consecutive days. Despite aggressive treatment, he continued to develop new blisters with extensive ocular and oral involvement. He rapidly became cachetic, bedbound and developed a chest infection. In the last 24 hours of life the erosions became more numerous and markedly haemorrhagic. He died in hospital 1 month after presentation. The postmortem identified bronchopneumonia as the cause of death. The para-aortic lymph nodes were grossly enlarged, the histopathology of which demonstrated lymphoplasmacytic lymphoma.

Comment

Paraneoplastic pemphigus (PNP) is a rare autoimmune bullous skin disease that occurs in association with an underlying neoplasm, usually a lymphoma. It was first described as a clinical and immunological entity separate from other forms of pemphigus in 1990.

PNP often presents clinically with a range of skin signs. In some cases a dermatosis suggestive of Stevens–Johnson syndrome is predominant, with erosions of the lips and oral cavity, conjunctivitis, genital involvement and target-like cutaneous lesions. Palms and soles are often involved. Lichenoid skin lesions are also well recognized in PNP, as are bullae and superficial erosions. In many cases, including our own, the eruption is polymorphic, with mucositis, erosions, blisters and lichenoid changes occurring simultaneously. The spectrum of clinical features leads to a broad differential diagnosis that includes erythema multiforme, lichen planus, lichenoid drug eruption, bullous pemphigoid and pemphigus.

The protean clinical findings are reflected in the range of histological features observed, including suprabasal acantholysis, subepidermal blistering, keratinocyte necrosis and lichenoid inflammation. Direct immunofluorescence demonstrates both intercellular and basement membrane zone deposition of IgG and complement (C3). Indirect immunofluorescence identifies circulating autoantibodies that bind to stratified as well as non-stratified epithelia (eg rat bladder and monkey oesophagus). Immunoprecitpitation and immunoblotting studies can yield antibodies reactive to some or all of the PNP proteins: 250 kDa (desmoplakin 1), 230 kDa (bullous pemphigoid antigen 1), 210 kDa (envoplakin), and 190 kDa (periplakin).

The presence of numerous target antigens in PNP has been explained by the phenomenon of epitope spreading. An initial lichenoid inflammatory process exposes hitherto covert autoantigens at the basement membrane zone and in the epidermis. Subsequent cell-mediated reactions may promote further autoimmunity, while humoral responses permit immunoglobulin reactivity to a range of epitopes (listed above), which are involved in keratinocyte cohesion and basement membrane zone adhesion.

There is no definitive treatment for PNP. However, powerful immunosuppressive therapies are usually required to control the disorder. The drugs commonly used include high-dose corticosteroids, intravenous immunoglobulins and mycophenolate mofetil. The anti-CD20 monoclonal antibody, rituximab has been reported to have clinical benefit on oral stomatitis recalcitrant to therapy. Despite aggressive chemotherapeutic interventions, the mortality remains poor at 90%.

Learning points

1. Paraneoplastic pemphigus (PNP) presents as a polymorphic mucocutaneous eruption in a patient with an underlying neoplasm, usually a lymphoma. Blisters, erosions, mucositis and lichenoid lesions are all recognized manifestations.
2. The histological findings from a skin biopsy reflect the spectrum of clinical features, including interface inflammation, suprabasal acantholysis and subepidermal blistering. Direct and indirect immunofluorescence studies are required for the diagnosis to be substantiated.
3. Despite aggressive immunosuppressive therapy, PNP has a very poor prognosis, with a 90% mortality rate.

Reference

Joly P, Richard C, Gilbert D et al. Sensitivity and specificity of clinical, histologic, and immunologic features in the diagnosis of paraneoplastic pemphigus. *J Am Acad Dermatol* 2000; 42: 619–26.

See also case numbers 1, 22.

Case 43
Abdominal pain, fever and acral purpura

History

A 36-year-old man was admitted acutely with a 3-day history of a fever, upper abdominal pain and widespread myalgia. The following day purpuric lesions were noted on the fingers and toes. A dermatology opinion was requested.

Clinical findings

The patient was febrile (38.8°C) and prostrate. There was upper abdominal tenderness. Examination of the hands and feet revealed numerous purpuric and pustular lesions of varying sizes (Figures 43a, b). Auscultation of the heart demonstrated a systolic murmur, loudest in the aortic area.

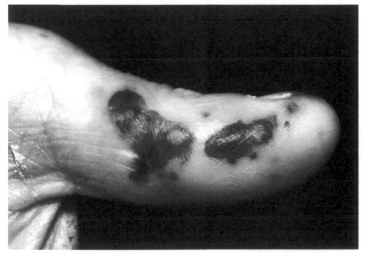

Figure 43a
Acute bacterial endocarditis.
Purpuric lesions on the thumb caused by emboli from an aortic valve vegetation.

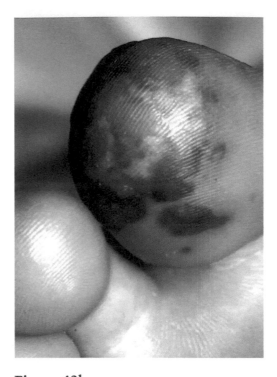

Figure 43b

Acute bacterial endocarditis.
Haemorrhagic and pustular lesions on the tip of the right great toe were caused by emboli containing Gram-positive cocci. Blood cultures isolated *Staphylococcus aureus*.

Investigations

Hb: 10.7 g/dl (11.5–15.5 g/dl), WCC: 4.29 × 10^9/l (4.0–11.0 × 10^9/l), plts: 46 × 10^9/l (150–450 × 10^9/l).

AST: 156 IU/l (10–50 IU/l), GGT: 198 IU/l (5–55 IU/l), bilirubin: 32 μmol/l (3–20 μmol/l), CRP: 347 mg/l (<5 mg/l) ESR: 77 mm/hr (1–10 mm/hr).

Urinalysis: blood +++, protein +++.

Skin histopathology: Biopsy of a purpuric lesion demonstrated the presence of emboli in vessels of the deep dermis. The emboli contained Gram-positive bacteria (Figure 43c).

Blood culture: There was growth of *Staphylococcus aureus*

Echocardiography: A bicuspid aortic valve was demonstrated with vegetations on the partially fused right and left coronary cusps. The vegetations prolapsed into the left ventricular outflow tract producing mild aortic regurgitation.

CT abdomen: There were renal and splenic embolic infarcts.

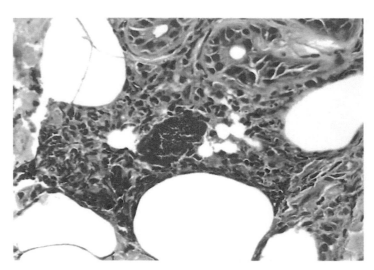

Figure 43c

Acute bacterial endocarditis.
Skin histopathology (H&E, high power). An embolus containing numerous Gram-positive bacteria is present in a deep dermal blood vessel.

Diagnosis

Acute bacterial endocarditis.

Treatment and progress

Further questioning revealed a history of intranasal cocaine abuse. A nasal swab grew *Staphylococcus aureus*, which was treated with topical fucidin ointment. The patient was commenced on intravenous flucloxacillin 2 g 4-hourly and gentamicin 120 mg 8-hourly. Initially, there was a good clinical response with resolution of fever, myalgia and abdominal pain and lowering of the CRP and ESR. Repeat echocardiographs suggested shrinkage of the vegetations. However, 3 weeks into treatment there was a sudden deterioration in the aortic valve function, and echocardiography demonstrated perforation of the non-coronary valve leaflet. The patient underwent surgical replacement of his aortic valve with a bioprosthesis (Figure 43d).

Comment

Infective endocarditis is a microbial infection of the endothelial lining of the heart producing a vegetation, usually on a valve. Subacute bacterial endocarditis (SBE) is typically caused by organisms, such as viridans streptococci, that possess only limited ability to infect other tissues, whereas acute bacterial endocarditis (ABE) is caused by pathogens, such as *S. aureus*, that are capable of causing invasive infection in other sites. In contrast to SBE, acute bacterial endocarditis typically evolves rapidly and aggressively over a period of days. Patients experience high fevers, rigors and prostration, usually leading to hospital admission. Embolic complications are common, with infarcts and metastatic infections developing in skin, internal viscera, bone or brain.

Patients with endocarditis may exhibit a variety of cutaneous signs, and, as in our case, a careful examination of the skin can indicate the diagnosis. Haemorrhagic skin infarcts are caused by emboli from vegetations present on the left side of the heart. If emboli are laden with bacteria then skin

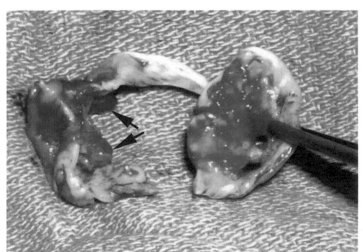

Figure 43d

Acute bacterial endocarditis.
The aortic valve was removed following a sudden deterioration in valvular function and replaced with a bioprosthetic valve. The arrows point to vegetations on the partially fused right and left coronary cusps. There are two perforations in the non-coronary cusp (being held by forceps).

sepsis may result, with the development of pustular lesions. Petechiae are caused by microembolization to small vessels in the skin and mucous membranes of the conjunctivae and hard palate. Splinter haemorrhages are also probably caused by microembolization to linear capillaries under the nail. Osler's nodes are painful tender erythematous nodules in the skin of the extremities, usually the pulp of the fingers. They are caused by inflammation around the site of lodgement of small infected emboli in distal arterioles. Janeway lesions are small (<5 mm), flat, non-tender red spots, irregular in outline, found on the palms and soles. Unlike petechiae, they are not haemorrhagic and blanch on pressure.

Blood culture is the critical investigation since it identifies the causative organism and guides antibiotic therapy. However, echocardiography is essential for the detection and monitoring of vegetations. Elevated CRP and ESR are usual; a normocytic anaemia, leucocytosis and thrombocytopenia are common. Proteinuria and microscopic haematuria are usually present.

The case fatality rate of bacterial endocarditis is approximately 20% and therefore close collaboration is needed between physician, microbiologist and cardiac surgeon. Any source of infection should be treated as soon as possible. Isolation of the organism allows the minimum bactericidal concentration (MBC) and minimum inhibitory concentration (MIC) of the antibiotic to be measured. Plasma antibiotic concentrations 4–8 times the MIC/MBC are recommended. Cardiac surgery is necessary in a substantial proportion of patients, especially in those with extensive valve damage, abscess formation and large, left-sided vegetations.

Learning points

1. The appearance of haemorrhagic infarcts on acral skin is suggestive of infective endocarditis and should direct the physician to a thorough examination of the heart.
2. Biopsy of a purpuric skin lesion can confirm the diagnosis of bacterial endocarditis by revealing bacteria-laden emboli within dermal vessels.
3. Acute bacterial endocarditis caused by *S. aureus* presents as a severe febrile illness often associated with disseminated embolic events and rapid valve destruction.

Reference

Hricak V, Kovacik J, Marks P et al. Aetiology and outcome in 53 cases of native valve Staphylococcal endocarditis. *Postgrad Med J* 1999; 75: 540–3.

See also case numbers 15, 30.

Case 44
Papules on the buttocks

History

A 44-year-old man presented with a 3-month history of an asymptomatic papular eruption on both buttocks. He was known to have hypertension but was otherwise well. His father had died in his forties of a heart attack.

Clinical findings

The patient was overweight. Examination of the skin revealed myriads of small, firm, monomorphic, yellowish papules on the buttocks (Figure 44a). Similar lesions were also observed on the upper arms and elbows.

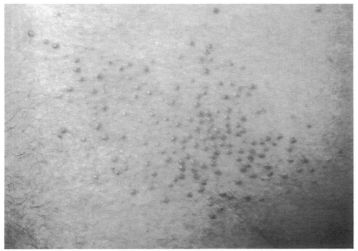

Figure 44a

Eruptive xanthomata.
There are multiple, firm, yellow papules present over the buttocks of this 44-year-old man with remnant particle disease (type III hyperlipidaemia).

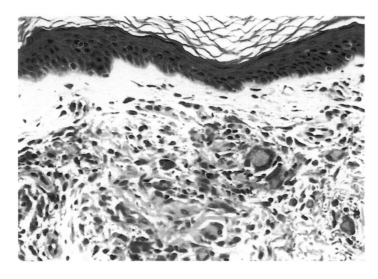

Figure 44b

Eruptive xanthomata.
Skin histopathology (H&E, medium power). An aggregate of foamy histiocytes and multinucleated giant cells is present in the dermis.

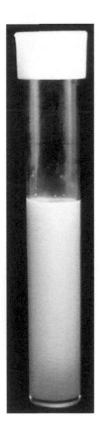

Figure 44c

Eruptive xanthomata.
Remnant particle disease (type III hyperlipidaemia). The patient's serum was found to be turbid from a high lipid content.

Investigations

Skin histopathology: Foamy histiocytes were seen throughout the dermis, with occasional giant cells. There was an associated perivascular inflammatory cell infiltrate (Figure 44b).

Serum cholesterol: 21.3 mmol/l (<5 mmol/l) (Figure 44c).

Serum triglyceride: 8.0 mmol/l (<2.3 mmol/l).

Diagnosis

Eruptive xanthomata.

Treatment and progress

Lipoprotein electrophoresis demonstrated that the patient had remnant particle disease (or type III hyperlipidaemia in the old terminology) secondary to familial dysbetalipoproteinaemia. He was commenced on a diet low

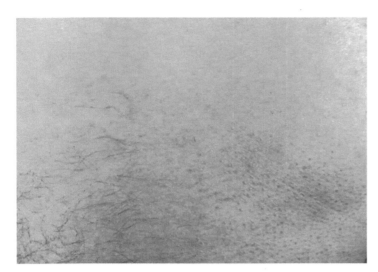

Figure 44d

Eruptive xanthomata.
Following treatment with appropriate lipid-lowering drugs and dietary manipulation the patient's eruptive xanthomata completely resolved.

in carbohydrate and cholesterol and advised to restrict alcohol consumption. In addition the lipid-lowering drugs bezafibrate and simvastatin were administered. Over the following year treatment resulted in normalization of the serum lipids and resolution of the xanthomata (Figure 44d).

Comment

Eruptive xanthomata generally develop rapidly over pressure points and on extensor surfaces and buttocks. Clinically, the lesions have a characteristically yellow colour, they are sometimes umbilicated and may possess an erythematous halo. As well as being associated with familial dysbetalipoproteinaemia, as in our case, eruptive xanthomata are also a feature of familial lipoprotein lipase deficiency and familial hypertriglyceridaemia. Eruptive xanthomata may occur as a secondary phenomenon in diabetes mellitus, in which insulin deficiency leads to an acquired lipoprotein lipase deficiency, producing combined hypercholesterolaemia or hypertriglyceridaemia.

Obese patients may develop these lesions because of an increased production of insulin resulting in the release of very low-density lipoprotein from the liver. Other exacerbating medical disorders include nephrotic syndrome, hypothyroidism, monoclonal gammopathies and alcoholism. Drug-induced hyperlipoproteinaemia has also been implicated in contributing to the formation of eruptive xanthomata; culprit drugs include oestrogens, corticosteroids and isotretinoin.

Learning points

1. It is important to recognize eruptive xanthomata since these lesions are a marker of significant hyperlipidaemia, which is associated with accelerated atherosclerosis.
2. The patient must be referred for appropriate evaluation and assessment of other cardiovascular risk factors.
3. Treatment of eruptive xanthomata involves treating the underlying hyperlipidaemia, which may either be a primary problem or secondary to another systemic disorder.

Histological examination of early skin lesions in eruptive xanthomatosis generally shows an infiltrate of cells and extravacular lipid deposits. In established lesions the lipidization of cells is more obvious, although foam cells are never as prominent as in the other forms of xanthoma.

Reference

Parker F. Xanthomas and hyperlipidemias. *J Am Acad Dermatol* 1985; 13: 1–30.

See also case numbers 19, 35.

Case 45
A non-healing crusted plaque in a child

History

A 6-year-old Algerian boy was referred with a 4-month history of a slowly growing crusted lesion on his right forearm. The general practitioner had prescribed flucloxacillin for presumed impetigo but there had been no improvement. The mother stated that the lesion had started at the site of an insect bite received whilst the family was staying in the Algerian desert. In addition, the patient's mother, brother and sister had also been bitten in the desert and all complained of persistent but smaller lesions at sites of insect bites.

Clinical findings

Examination of the boy revealed a 5 cm diameter crusted, indurated red plaque on the dorsal aspect of the right wrist (Figure 45a). There was no regional lymphadenopathy. The patient's mother had a red crusted nodule on a finger while the boy's siblings had similar solitary nodules on the left arm and right leg respectively (Figure 45b).

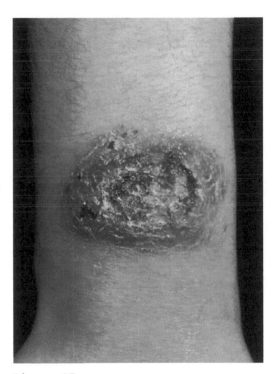

Figure 45a

Old World leishmaniasis.
An inflammatory, crusted plaque on the dorsal aspect of the right forearm of a 6-year-old boy who was bitten by a sandfly in Algeria 4 months earlier.

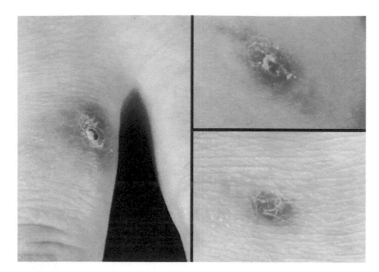

Figure 45b

Old World leishmaniasis.
The boy's family members also had persistent red, crusted nodules at the site of insect bites acquired at the same time in Algeria. *Left:* Mother, finger. *Upper right:* Brother, left arm. *Lower right:* Sister, right knee. All lesions were leishmaniasis.

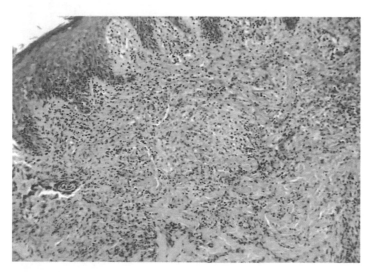

Figure 45c

Old World leishmaniasis.
Skin histopathology (H&E, low power). The epidermis is acanthotic with an underlying inflammatory cell infiltrate present throughout the dermis.

Investigations

Skin histopathology: The epidermis was acanthotic while within the dermis there was an intense inflammatory cell infiltrate composed of histiocytes, plasma cells, lymphocytes and occasional eosinophils (Figure 45c). The histiocytes contained numerous Leishman–Donovan bodies (Figure 45d).

Skin culture: *Leishmania major* was cultured.

Diagnosis

Cutaneous Old World leishmaniasis.

Treatment and progress

The children were given oral itraconazole 4 mg/kg/day. The mother received intralesional sodium stibogluconate every 2 weeks. After 2 months of therapy the lesions had resolved in all the family members.

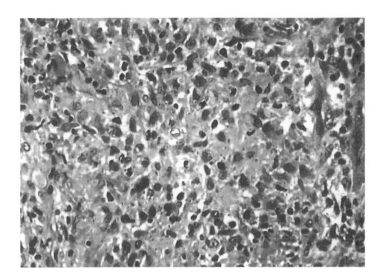

Figure 45d

Old World leishmaniasis.
Skin histopathology (H&E, high power). Numerous organisms are present in the cytoplasm of macrophages (Leishman–Donovan bodies).

Comment

Leishmaniasis is a protozoal disease with a wide spectrum of clinical manifestations, including cutaneous and visceral forms. It is caused by species of the genus *Leishmania*, transmitted through the bite of the sandfly. Old World leishmaniasis is found in the dry regions of North Africa, East Africa, Afghanistan, India, the Middle East and the Mediterranean Coast (which includes common holiday destinations such as Spain, southern France, Italy and Greece). The species responsible are *L. major* in the Middle East and North Africa, *L. tropica* in India, Afghanistan and the Mediterranean Coast and *L. aethiopica* in Ethiopia, Yemen and East Africa.

The amastigote form of *Leishmaniasis* is ingested by the female sandfly whilst feeding from an infected mammal. The parasite then develops into the promastigote form in the midgut of the sandfly and multiplies. The mature promastigotes migrate to the proboscis and are inoculated into a new mammalian host. Once introduced, promastigotes are taken up by, and multiply within, histiocytes and monocytes (Leishman–Donovan bodies). After an incubation period ranging from a few days to several months, infection is recognized immunologically and a cutaneous lesion appears. Generally, one or more lesions occur on exposed skin, usually in a child. The face, neck and arms are the commonest targets. As in our case, all members of a family may develop lesions and recall receiving bites simultaneously.

The natural history of cutaneous lesions in Old World leishmaniasis varies according to the species involved. However, the sequence of nodule, crusting, ulceration and spontaneous healing is common to all. Typically, *L. major* infections commence as a red nodule at the site of inoculation with the subsequent development of an overlying crust. The crust may persist or fall away exposing an ulcer. The lesion expands over the next 3 months, reaching a diameter of 3–6 cm. Healing generally occurs over the following 6 months, leaving a scar.

The diagnosis may be made on clinical grounds in those returning from endemic areas. Identification of the parasite may be made on a smear from lesional material or by the identification of Leishman–Donovan

Learning points

1. The diagnosis of Old World leishmaniasis should be considered in a patient presenting with a non-healing crusted lesion on exposed skin who has a recent history of travel to an endemic area (North Africa, East Africa, Afghanistan, India, the Middle East and the Mediterranean Coast).
2. A skin biopsy must be performed to establish the diagnosis. Material should be sent for routine histopathology and for microbiological analysis and culture.
3. Examine other family members for lesions of leishmaniasis if they have also been to the same endemic area.

Occasionally, polymerase chain reaction (PCR) analysis for leishmanial DNA may be needed to make the diagnosis.

The lesions of cutaneous leishmaniasis usually heal spontaneously but with scarring; therefore the object of treatment is to maximize the cosmetic outcome. Pentavalent antimonials are the drugs of choice and can be given intralesionally or systemically. Azoles, such as itraconazole and ketaconazole, also appear be effective, while cryotherapy or excision may be used for small lesions.

bodies on histopathology. Culture of biopsy material on Novy–MacNeal–Nicolle medium will help to identify the species.

Reference

Faber WR, Oskam L, van Gool T et al. Value of diagnostic techniques for cutaneous leishmaniasis. *J Am Acad Dermatol* 2003; 49: 70–4.

See also case number 23.

Case 46
A rash on the face, upper back and hands

History

A 32-year-old woman presented with a rash on her face. She complained of sore and itchy reddening of the skin of the forehead and temples. The eruption extended to the hairline and into the scalp, where it was associated with hair loss. After several weeks a similar eruption appeared on her shoulders and on the backs of the hands. She was otherwise well.

Clinical findings

There was an erythematous, non-scaly, macular dermatosis involving the periphery of the face, the hairline and the lateral neck (Figure 46a). Involvement of the scalp was accompanied by non-scarring alopecia. On the upper back there was an extensive area of macular, violaceous erythema (Figure 46b). Examination of the hands revealed inflammatory papules on the dorsal aspects of the fingers with particular prominence over the finger joints (Figure 46c). There was erythema of the nail folds with visible capillaries and dystrophic cuticles (Figure 46d).

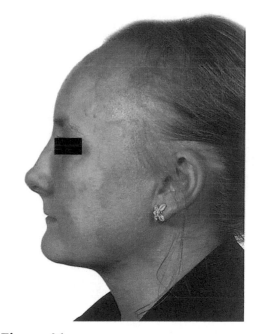

Figure 46a

Dermatomyositis.
This 32-year-old woman presented with an erythematous macular eruption that affected the forehead, cheeks, hairline and scalp. Scalp involvement was characterized by non-scarring alopecia.

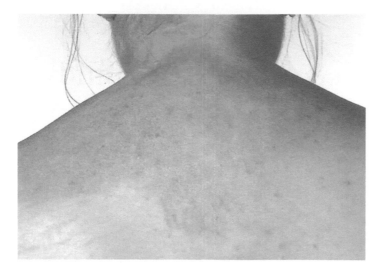

Figure 46b

Dermatomyositis.
Macular, violaceous erythema was
present over the upper back and neck
(shawl sign).

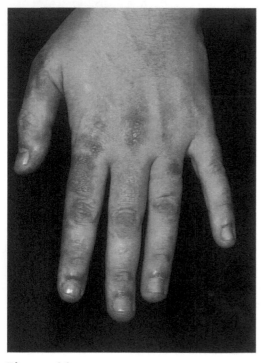

Figure 46c

Dermatomyositis.
Violaceous, shiny papules were present on
the dorsal aspects of the fingers,
particularly over the knuckles and
interphalangeal joints. This is Gottron's
sign.

Investigations

Hb:12.4 g/dl (11.5–15.5 g/dl), WCC: 7.37 ×
10^9/l (4.0–11.0 × 10^9/l), plts: 260 × 10^9/l (150–
450 × 10^9/l). ESR: 6 mm/hr (1–10 mm/hr).

U&E: normal, LFT: normal.

ANA: negative, ENA: negative.

Rheumatoid factor: negative.

Creatine kinase: 121 IU/l (0–150 IU/l).

Skin histopathology: There was hyperkeratosis, mild epidermal atrophy and an interface
lymphocytic infiltrate at the dermo–epidermal junction with basal vacuolar degeneration and colloid body formation (Figure 46e).

Diagnosis

Dermatomyositis.

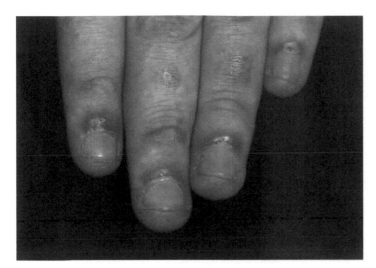

Figure 46d

Dermatomyositis.
There was erythema of the proximal nail folds with visible capillaries. The cuticles were dystrophic.

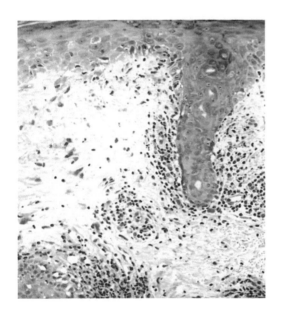

Figure 46e

Dermatomyositis.
Skin histopathology (H&E, medium power). There is an interface lymphocytic infiltrate with basal vacuolar degeneration and colloid body formation, occurring most prominently around a hair follicle. These changes are indistinguishable from lupus erythematosus.

Treatment and progress

Initially, a diagnosis of dermatomyositis sine myositis (amyotrophic dermatomyositis) was made and the patient was treated with topical clobetasol propionate 0.05% and oral hydroxychloroquine. However, over the ensuing 3 months the disorder continued to evolve with the development of swelling and redness of the eyelids, dysphagia, dysphonia and weakness of the limb musculature (Figure 46f). The diagnosis was therefore revized to classical dermatomyositis. She found it increasingly difficult climbing stairs and getting in and out of her car. Repeated investigations revealed elevated inflammatory markers (ESR: 79 mm/hr) and muscle enzymes (creatine kinase: 430 IU/l). Although a muscle biopsy did not demonstrate inflammation, polymyositis was apparent clinically and investigations were undertaken to exclude an underlying neoplasm. The following were normal or negative: chest x-ray; CT scan of neck, thorax, abdomen and pelvis; mammography, upper gastrointestinal endoscopy; faecal occult blood analysis; nasopharyngeal examination; cervical smear cytology; serum carcinoembryonic antigen, alpha-fetoprotein, CA-125 and CA-19-9.

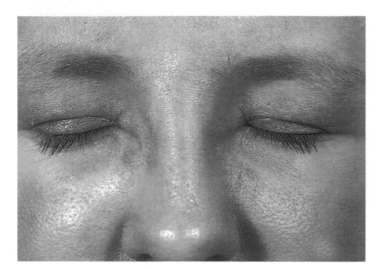

Figure 46f

Dermatomyositis.
As the DM worsened with symptomatic polymyositis, periorbital involvement became evident. The eyelids became oedematous and developed a blue-red (heliotrope) erythema.

The patient failed to respond to prednisolone and methotrexate and so was treated with intravenous methyl-prednisolone 500 mg on 3 consecutive days and intravenous immunoglobulin at a dose of 2 g/kg monthly for 3 consecutive months. Following high-dose immunosuppressive therapy the myositis resolved completely with loss of muscle symptoms and normalization of the serum creatine kinase. There was, however, an incomplete response of the cutaneous features and so she was commenced on azathioprine, eventually tolerating a dose of 175 mg/day. Six months after initiation of azathioprine there was clearance of the facial erythema, loss of the eyelid oedema and hair regrowth.

Comment

Dermatomyositis (DM) is a disorder in which autoimmune inflammatory injury occurs in the skin and striated muscle. As in our case, the skin disease commonly precedes muscle involvement and affected individuals may display cutaneous features alone for up to 6 months before the onset of polymyositis. Occasionally the dermatosis of DM occurs in isolation, when it is known as dermatomyositis sine myositis (or amyotrophic DM).

The clinical picture is variable; however, the classical cutaneous manifestations of DM include a characteristic blue–red (heliotrope) erythema of the eyelids accompanied by periorbital oedema, while examination of the hands reveals violaceous papules on the dorsal aspect of the fingers, particularly over the proximal nail folds, joints and knuckles (Gottron's papules). Prominent periungual erythema with visible dilated capillary loops is typical and is associated with ragged dystrophic cuticles. The facial rash often involves the upper cheeks, forehead and temples. Macular erythema may also extend to the arms, posterior shoulders and neck (shawl sign) and the V of the chest. Involvement of the hairline and scalp, as in our patient, is recognized and is associated with non-scarring alopecia. A wide variety of other skin changes have been described, including bullous lesions, urticaria, ulceration, photosensitivity, flagellate erythema and psoriasiform eruptions. Healing lesions can leave areas of telangiectatic erythema with atrophy and dyspigmentation (poikiloderma).

The myositis of DM usually presents as symmetrical weakness of the proximal musculature of the legs and arms resulting in difficulty with routine activities of daily living. Tenderness and pain in the affected muscle groups is common. Uncontrolled, progressive myositis can result in involvement of the bulbar and respiratory muscles with potentially life-threatening sequelae.

Diagnosis of DM is based on the recognition of typical cutaneous signs in the presence of an inflammatory myositis. Muscle involvement can be demonstrated by elevated muscle enzymes, diagnostic electromyographic changes and patterns of muscle inflammation on biopsy. However, myositic inflammation can be highly focal and tissue sampling may not reveal diagnostic changes, as in our case. Elevated antinuclear antibody (ANA) levels are seen in approximately 70% of patients with DM, while antibodies to Jo-1 are demonstrable in 20% of cases. Other significant investigations include the ESR, which is elevated in roughly 50% of cases of DM but does not correlate closely with disease activity. Histopathology of involved skin tends to demonstrate lupus erythematosus-like changes with an interface dermatitis and vacuolar degeneration of the basal keratinocytes.

In certain circumstances DM is associated with an underlying neoplasm; studies have demonstrated a relative risk for malignancy in DM patients of up to 26.0. Women with DM appear to have a specific susceptibility to developing ovarian carcinoma. In patients with an associated malignancy the DM is less responsive to systemic corticosteroid therapy. However, definitive therapy for the underlying cancer can result in resolution of the DM.

Systemic immunosuppressive therapy is usually required to control the cutaneous and myopathic features of DM. A standard combination is oral prednisolone with or without another immunosuppressive agent, such as methotrexate or azathioprine. Patients who do not respond to oral therapy may require, as with our case, intravenous methylprednisolone or high-dose intravenous immunoglobulin.

Learning points

1. Cutaneous signs of dermatomyositis (DM) may precede clinical evidence of myositis by many months. Typical skin signs include: erythema and swelling of the eyelids, violaceous papules on the dorsal aspect of the fingers, periungual erythema, and a macular rash on the face, arms and V of the chest. Unusual skin signs include: alopecia, bullous lesions, ulceration, flagellate erythema and poikiloderma.
2. Prior to treatment the patient should be evaluated to assess the extent of systemic involvement and the presence of an underlying malignancy.
3. The skin involvement and myositis of DM may respond variably and independently to systemic immunosuppressive therapy.

Reference

Sontheimer RD. Dermatomyositis: an overview of recent progress with emphasis on dermatologic aspects. *Dermatol Clin* 2002; 20: 387–408.

See also case numbers 18, 26.

Case 47
A large vascular tumour in an HIV-positive man

History

A 34-year-old HIV-positive Ugandan man presented with a large tumour involving the skin and subcutaneous tissue of the left thigh. He also complained of pain in the left sternoclavicular joint. The cutaneous lesion had been previously excised, but had rapidly regrown.

Clinical features

The patient was febrile (37.9°C). There was an 8 cm × 4 cm red, lobulated, dome-shaped tumour present on the lateral aspect of the left thigh (Figure 47a). The surface was ulcerated and oozed a sero-sanguinous fluid. The surrounding skin was firm and indurated. Lymphadenopathy was palpable in the left groin. There was tenderness over the left clavicle.

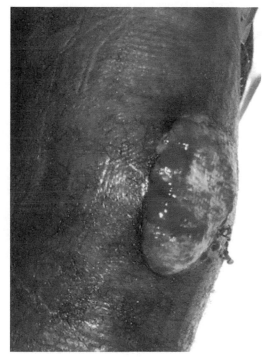

Figure 47a

Bacillary angiomatosis.
There is a large, solitary, dome-shaped vascular tumour arising from the skin of the left thigh in this HIV-positive man. The surface was ulcerated and bled easily.

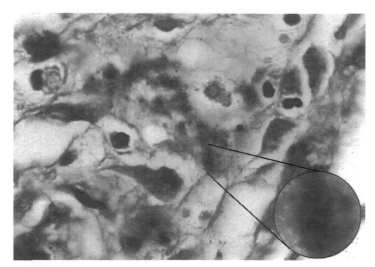

Figure 47b

Bacillary angiomatosis.
Skin histopathology (Giemsa, high power). There are clumps of eosinophilic granular material within the stroma adjacent to endothelial cells. They can be seen more clearly when magnified further (*inset*). These are aggregates of *Bartonella* bacilli.

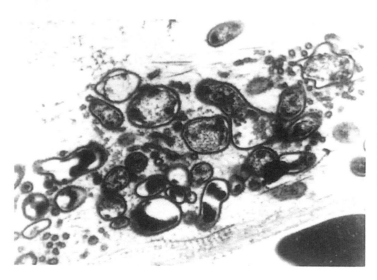

Figure 47c

Bacillary angiomatosis.
Electron microscopy of skin biopsy. There is a cluster of bacilli in the extracellular matrix. The bacilli measure 1–1.5 µm long and 0.25–0.5 µm in diameter. Each microorganism is surrounded by a 30–40 nm thick trilaminar wall that is characteristic of the vegetative forms of Gram-negative bacteria.

Investigations

Hb: 8.5 g/dl (11.5–15.5 g/dl), WCC: 3.4 × 10⁹/l (4.0–11.0 × 10⁹/l), lymphs: 0.24 × 10⁹/l(1.3–4.0 × 10⁹/l), plts: 174 × 10⁹/l (150–450 × 10⁹/l). ESR: 84 mm/hr (1–10 mm/hr).

CD4 count: <20 cells/mm³.

U&E: normal, LFT: normal.

TPHA: negative.

Plain x-rays: Multiple lytic lesions were present in the medial end of the left clavicle.

Skin histopathology: The lesion consisted of vascular lobules composed of rounded aggregates of capillaries. In places the endothelial cells possessed an epithelioid appearance. There was a florid inflammatory infiltrate in the stroma containing numerous neutrophils. Clumps of granular purple material were seen interstitially between vessels (Figure 47b), which, when viewed with electron microscopy, were demonstrated to be bacilli (Figure 47c).

Diagnosis

Bacillary angiomatosis.

Treatment and progress

The patient was treated with intravenous erythromycin 1 g 4 times a day. After 7 days there was a marked reduction in the size of the tumour and improvement in the exudate. He was then switched to oral azithromycin 2 g daily, and after 4 months of treatment the lesion had completely resolved. The bony pain also settled with antibiotic therapy.

This patient presented in the era prior to the introduction of highly active anti-retroviral therapy (HAART) and although his bacillary angiomatosis was treated successfully he thereafter developed further infectious illnesses and died 10 months later from disseminated *Mycobacterium avium intracellulare* infection.

Comment

Bacillary angiomatosis (BA) is a rare angioproliferative disorder caused by infection with *Bartonella henselae* or occasionally *B. quintana*. It tends to occur in immunosuppressed patients, most commonly in those with AIDS, but also in transplant recipients and patients with leukaemia. BA is usually characterized by the development of multiple, widely disseminated, angiomatous papules 2–10 mm in diameter. Atypical presentations include indurated hyperpigmented plaques, skin-coloured subcutaneous nodules, violaceous plaques and, as in our case, a solitary vascular tumour. Constitutional signs and symptoms may accompany the appearance of skin lesions; fever, malaise, lymphadenopathy and weight loss are common. Extracutaneous involvement with BA is not unusual, and biopsy-proven lesions have been demonstrated in the liver, spleen, bone marrow and respiratory tract. Skeletal involvement is also well recognized, usually presenting with focal bone pain, as with our patient, and identified radiologically by the presence lytic lesions.

B. henselae is a small, Gram-negative, rod-shaped bacterium, which can cause cat scratch disease as well as BA. The domestic cat is the main reservoir of *B. henselae* and several studies have established an association between the incidence of BA and exposure to cats. Following bacterial inoculation, *B. henselae* initially invades erythrocytes and thereafter, in a susceptible host, can infect and activate vascular endothelium. Angiomatosis is mediated by uncontrolled angiogenic signalling, which is most probably driven by the presence of *Bartonella* bacilli. Histology of a BA lesion demonstrates a lobulated vasoproliferation, the vessels being lined by plump epithelioid endothelial cells. An accompanying inflammatory cell infiltrate is usual and neutrophils are particularly numerous in deeper lesions. Aggregates of *Bartonella* organisms may be seen as minute clumps of eosinophilic granular material. These can be identified more clearly using Warthin–Starry silver stain or with electron microscopy.

The clinical differential diagnosis of BA includes pyogenic granuloma, Kaposi sarcoma, haemangioma and angiokeratoma; therefore the definitive diagnosis should be made histologically. Treatment of BA is with prolonged courses of antibiotics: erythromycin, azithromycin and doxycycline are first-line therapies. The optimal duration of treatment is not clear; however, many cases show complete resolution after 8 weeks of antibiotic therapy.

Learning points

1. Bacillary angiomatosis (BA) is a vasoproliferative disease occurring in immunocompromised individuals caused by infection with *Bartonella henselae*. Infection of immunocompetent patients with the same organism can cause cat scratch disease.
2. Clinically, BA is usually characterized by multiple, disseminated, small angiomatous papules. However, atypical presentations include plaques, nodules and vascular tumours. Lymphadenopathy and systemic involvement are common.
3. Diagnosis is made following a skin biopsy. *Bartonella* bacilli can be seen in the biopsy with the use of special stains or electron microscopy.

Reference

Gasquet S, Maurin M, Bronqui P et al. Bacillary angiomatosis in immunocompromized patients. *AIDS* 1998; 12; 1793–1803.

See also case number 40.

Case 48
Linear blisters and pigmentation in a baby girl

History

A baby girl born at full term developed a vesicular eruption on the legs at 3 weeks of age. She was otherwise well. Viral and bacterial cultures of skin swabs were negative. The dermatosis persisted and at 2 months she developed linear hyperpigmentation on her legs and further vesicles on her abdomen. On close questioning the mother thought that she had also suffered from a blistering skin problem during infancy.

Clinical findings

Examination of the skin revealed a polymorphic eruption. On the inner aspect of the left thigh there were numerous papulovesicles, some arranged in a linear pattern (Figure 48a). On the posterior aspect of the right thigh there was linear hyperpigmentation. On the left lower leg there was speckled hyperpigmentation that ran in a linear distribution down to the heel (Figure 48b). On the right flank there was an erythematous, wavy streak that followed Blaschko's lines.

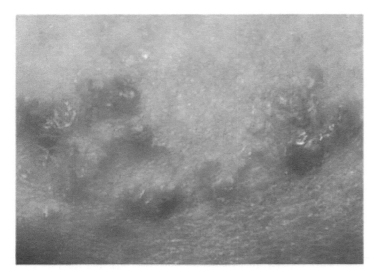

Figure 48a

Incontinentia pigmenti.
Vesicular lesions arranged in a linear configuration on the inner aspect of the left thigh of a 3-week-old baby girl. This eruption is consistent with the first, inflammatory stage of incontinentia pigmenti.

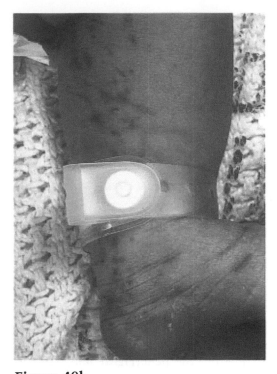

Figure 48b

Incontinentia pigmenti.
Speckled hyperpigmentation in a linear
distribution on the left lower leg
developed following the resolution of
inflammatory lesions. Hyperpigmented
stage of incontinentia pigmenti.

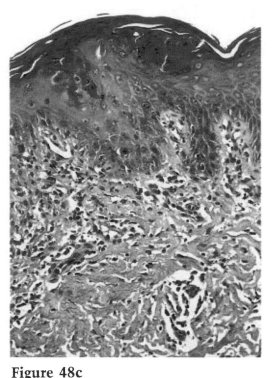

Figure 48c

Incontinentia pigmenti.
Skin histopathology (H&E, medium
power). Biopsy of a pigmented lesion
demonstrated epidermal acanthosis
containing numerous dyskeratotic
keratinocytes and an underlying
inflammatory cell infiltrate with pigment-
laden macrophages.

Investigations

Skin histopathology: Biopsy of a vesicle
revealed a prominent superficial dermal
infiltrate of eosinophils with epidermal
exocytosis, eosinophilic spongiosis and intraepidermal vesicle formation. Biopsy of a
pigmented lesion demonstrated an acanthotic
epidermis containing numerous dyskeratotic
cells with a mixture of inflammatory cells
and pigment-laden macrophages in the underlying papillary dermis (Figure 48c).

Diagnosis

Incontinentia pigmenti.

Treatment and progress

During infancy, the eruption settled, leaving
first hyperpigmentation and then scarring,
most prominently on the legs. The patient

suffered two grand mal seizures during her childhood but was not considered to have any significant neurological pathology. Her deciduous dentition was shed late and a number of her permanent teeth were conical in shape.

Examination of the mother's legs demonstrated a number of vertically-aligned linear scars.

Comment

Incontinentia pigmenti (IP) is a genodermatosis inherited as an X-linked dominant disorder that is usually lethal prenatally in males. In affected females, the disease presents in the neonatal period and is characterized by evolving, polymorphic skin lesions, by other ectodermal abnormalities, and by variable involvement of the eyes and central nervous system. There may be a history of miscarriages and neonatal rashes in the female line. The mother should be examined carefully for residual clinical signs indicative of active disease in infancy. The skin lesions follow Blaschko's lines (reflecting the somatic mutation due to X-chromosome inactivation in females) and occur in four sequential stages: (1) inflammatory, (2) verrucous, (3) hyperpigmented and (4) scarred. However, not all stages develop in every case.

The first stage begins at approximately 2 weeks of life and inflammatory lesions can continue to develop until 4–6 months of age. Vesicles and erythematous patches appear that follow a linear configuration. Histologically, there is eosinophilic infiltration into the epidermis, producing spongiosis. Subsequently, verrucous lesions occur between 2 and 6 months of age. As the vesicular and warty lesions resolve, areas of hyperpigmentation remain. The pigmentation fades spontaneously leaving pale, hairless anhidrotic scars. Recurrence of inflammatory lesions several months or years after their initial resolution has been reported and tends to occur after an unconnected febrile illness.

The hair abnormalities seen in IP occur in approximately 50% of patients and are subtle, usually manifesting as sparse, lacklustre hair. In the adult, areas of scarring alopecia radiating from the vertex of the scalp can be a residual sign of IP. Nail abormalities range from minimal ridging to a severe, disgfiguring dystrophy. Dental abnormalities include delayed eruption, hypodontia and abnormally shaped crowns. Ocular abnormalities, including strabismus, refractive error and proliferative retinopathy, are seen in up to 40% cases. Only 5% of patients have severe neurological problems. However, up to 15% of cases have a related central nervous system disorder, with epilepsy being the commonest association.

IP has recently been ascribed to mutations in the *NEMO* gene (NF-κB Essential MOdulator). The mutated *NEMO* gene encodes a non-functional protein, unable to activate the NF-κB pathway. Cells in which the mutant X chromosome remains active are devoid of NF-κB activation and become more sensitive to apoptosis and hyperproliferation. In the majority of cases a gene rearrangement truncates the *NEMO* gene, causing loss of function. It is therefore unable to activate the transcription factor, which is essential to many immune, inflammatory and apoptotic pathways.

Learning points

1. Incontinentia pigmenti (IP) presents shortly after birth in female infants (being inherited in an X-linked dominant fashion) with vesicles that evolve into verrucous, hyperpigmented and ultimately scarred lesions that follow Blaschko's lines. A skin biopsy will support the clinical diagnosis.
2. IP is associated with ocular and central nervous system problems; therefore at diagnosis the patient should undergo ophthalmological and neurological examinations.
3. IP is caused by mutations affecting the *NEMO* gene that cause impaired activation of the transcription factor NF-κB.

Reference

Smahi A, Courtois G, Vabres P et al. Genomic rearrangement in *NEMO* impairs NF-κB activation and is a cause of incontinentia pigmenti. *Nature* 2000; 405: 466–72.

See also case number 27.

Case 49
Gradual coarse wrinkling of the skin

History

A 33-year-old woman from Barbados presented with progressive changes to her skin. Over the previous 15 years she had noticed that the skin of her neck, flanks, armpits and groins had gradually developed a lumpy texture with coarse wrinkling. She was otherwise well. She had been adopted and so no family history was obtainable.

Clinical findings

The skin of the trunk was thrown into coarse folds with exaggeration of the normal creases (Figure 49a). On palpation, the skin had a papular, indurated texture. Examination of the neck revealed yellow papules with prominent skin wrinkling (Figure 49b). Pendulous, lax folds were present in the axillae and groins (Figure 49c). Bilateral angioid streaks were present on fundoscopy (Figure 49d). The blood pressure was 190/105.

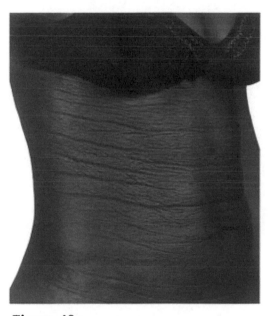

Figure 49a

Pseudoxanthoma elasticum.
The skin of the trunk appeared excessively wrinkled with exaggeration of the normal creases.

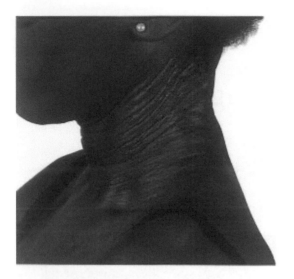

Figure 49b

Pseudoxanthoma elasticum.
The skin of the neck is characterized by the presence of coarse transverse folds. Closer examination revealed multiple yellow papules.

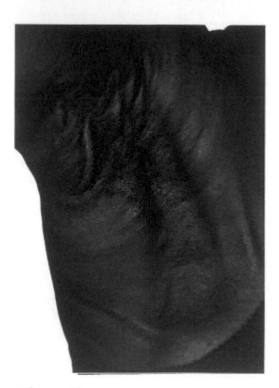

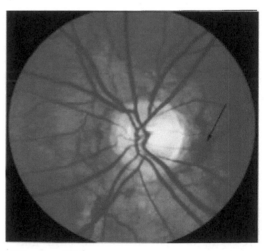

Figure 49d

Pseudoxanthoma elasticum.
Fundoscopic examination demonstrated angioid streaks (arrowed), which are fissures in Bruch's membrane of the retina and appear as angulated red lines, thicker than retinal vessels, radiating from the optic disc.

Figure 49c

Pseudoxanthoma elasticum.
Redundant, pendulous folds of lax skin were present in the axillae. Similar changes were observed in the groins.

Investigations

Skin histopathology: Biopsy of a yellow papule from the neck revealed that irregular aggregates of clumped, thickened, elastic fibres present in the papillary and reticular dermis. A von Kossa stain demonstrated calcification of the abnormal elastic fibres.

Diagnosis

Pseudoxanthoma elasticum.

Treatment and progress

The patient was underwent a full cardiological assessment, which demonstrated some left ventricular hypertrophy. She was commenced on anti-hypertensive medication, which normalized her blood pressure. The patient was advised to cease smoking. She was kept under regular review in the departments of dermatology, cardiology and ophthalmology.

Comment

Pseudoxanthoma elasticum (PXE) is a rare, hereditary, multi-system connective tissue disorder that is characterized by progressive calcification of abnormal elastic fibres in the skin, blood vessels and Bruch's membrane of the retina. It has an incidence of 1–2:160 000 with a female-to-male ratio of 2:1 and affects all races.

The characteristic initial skin lesions are small yellow papules that coalesce into plaques with a 'plucked chicken' or 'cobblestone' appearance, particularly prominent on the neck and at flexural sites. Changes usually commence in childhood and thereafter progress to redundant skin folds in the major flexures.

The systemic effects of PXE are the consequence of calcification of other organs rich in elastic connective tissue, including the retina and cardiovascular system. Angioid streaks, caused by cracking of Bruch's membrane of the retina, are seen in 85% of patients with PXE. Other ocular complications include retinal haemorrhages. The formation of atheroma and increased vascular fragility can lead to stroke or myocardial infarction, while involvement of renal arteries can induce hypertension. Rupture of superficial vessels in the gastrointestinal tract is a common source of bleeding and anaemia in PXE. There may be an increased risk of miscarriage in the first trimester in women.

Recent advances in the genetics of PXE have identified multiple defects in the *ABCC6* gene on chromosome 16p13.1 encoding for the MRP6 protein, a transmembrane transporter. Different genetic types of PXE have been identified with differing clinical phenotypes ranging from severe atheroma and degenerative retinopathy with early blindness (dominant and recessive type I), to moderate disease with features of Marfan's syndrome (dominant II) to mild disease with no systemic complications (recessive II).

The course of the disease may be improved with early diagnosis and by introducing a diet low in fat and calcium, avoiding smoking and treating the associated hypertension.

Learning points

1. Pseudoxanthoma elasticum (PXE) is a disease affecting the elastic connective tissue and resulting in both cutaneous and systemic pathology. Ocular complications can result in blindness, whilst vascular involvement can be life-threatening.
2. A skin biopsy will strengthen the clinical diagnosis by demonstrating calcification of clumped and thickened dermal elastic fibres. These connective tissue ultrastructural changes are better delineated with electron microscopy.
3. Early diagnosis and instigation of measures to limit systemic progression may reduce morbidity and mortality.

Reference

Hu X, Bergen S et al. *ABCC6*/MRP6 mutations: further insight into the molecular pathology of pseudoxanthoma elasticum. *Eur J Hum Genet* 2003; 11: 215–224.

See also case number 5.

Case 50
Breathlessness and widespread cutaneous necrosis

History

A 32-year-old Nigerian woman presented with a 2-week history of worsening breathlessness, headache and a rash. She also complained of a cough, productive of blood-stained sputum. She was known to have poorly controlled asthma and rhinitis. She was admitted acutely and transferred immediately to the intensive care unit (ICU). On the ICU she was found to have extensive purpura, and a dermatology opinion was requested.

Clinical findings

On examination, the patient was febrile (38.6°C), orientated but drowsy. She was tachycardic and hypotensive. Examination of the skin demonstrated numerous purpuric lesions with some larger areas of cutaneous necrosis scattered over her trunk and limbs (Figures 50a, b). A number of the lesions demonstrated a stellate configuration; others were bullous. Although the purpura was suggestive of meningococcal septicaemia, there was no clinical evidence of meningism.

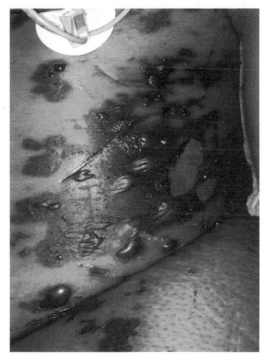

Figure 50a

Churg–Strauss syndrome.
This patient with poorly controlled asthma and rhinitis was admitted to the ICU with respiratory distress and large purpuric lesions on the flanks. Some lesions were blistering; in other areas there was epithelial denudation.

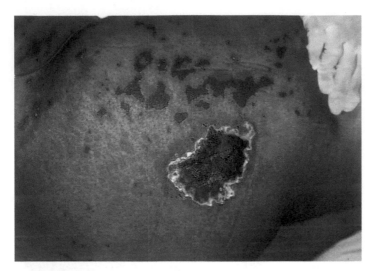

Figure 50b

Churg–Strauss syndrome.
Some of the purpuric lesions (upper) demonstrated a livedoid or stellate appearance. In other areas the vasculitis produced full-thickness skin necrosis (lower lesion).

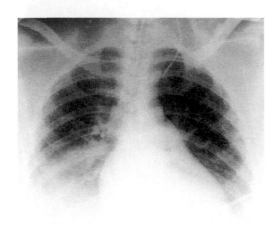

Figure 50c

Churg–Strauss syndrome.
Chest radiograph. There are diffuse interstitial infiltrates through both lung fields. These changes are typical in advanced pulmonary CSS.

Investigations

Hb: 7.7 g/dl (11.5–15.5 g/dl), WCC: 11.3 × 10^9/l (4.0–11.0 × 10^9/l), eos: 4.69 × 10^9/l (0–0.4 10^9/l), PMN: 4.9 × 10^9/l (2.0–5.0 × 10^9/l), plts: 157 × 10^9/l (150–450 × 10^9/l).

D-dimer: 1728 μg/l (<200 μg/l).

ESR: 104 mm/hr (1–10 mm/hr).

Chest x-ray: This showed extensive bilateral interstitial infiltrates (Figure 50c).

Lumbar puncture: normal.

Blood culture: negative

ANA: negative, pANCA: positive.

Skin histopathology: Biopsy of a purpuric lesion demonstrated a widespread small and medium vessel vasculitis. The vascular infiltrate was composed predominantly of eosinophils (Figures 50d, e).

Diagnosis

Churg–Strauss syndrome.

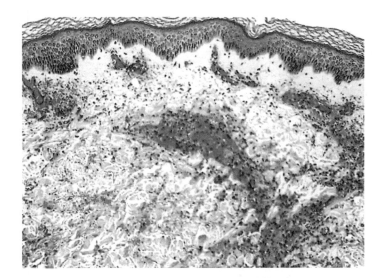

Figure 50d

Churg–Strauss syndrome.
Skin histopathology (H&E, low power). There is an intense perivascular inflammatory cell infiltrate involving small and medium-sized vessels throughout the full thickness of the dermis.

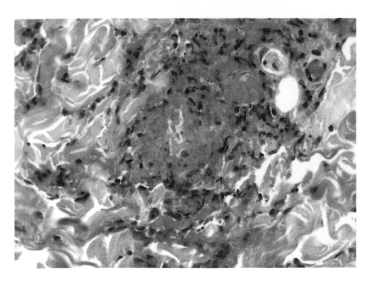

Figure 50e

Churg–Strauss syndrome.
Skin histopathology (H&E, high power). There is vasculitis with fibrin necrosis and intravascular thrombus. The vascular infiltrate is predominantly composed of eosinophils.

Treatment and progress

Since the eruption was suggestive of meningococcal septicaemia (purpura fulminans), the patient received broad-spectrum antibiotics. However, once bacterial sepsis had been excluded and eosinophilic vasculitis identified, immunosuppressive therapy with methylprednisolone and cyclophosphamide was instituted. Shortly after transfer to the ICU she developed severe bronchospasm with respiratory exhaustion, necessitating intubation and ventilation. She also became acidotic and oliguric, requiring haemofiltration and inotrope support. One week later she developed an acute abdomen and her clinical state deteriorated. Blood cultures grew a vancomycin-resistant *Enterococcus*. Sixteen days after presentation she died of peritonitis.

Comment

Churg–Strauss syndrome (CSS) is a multi-system disease characterized by asthma, eosinophilia and vasculitis. The diagnosis can be made if four of the following criteria are met: asthma, eosinophilia (>10% of the total white cell count), neuropathy, migratory pulmonary infiltrates on chest radiograph, paranasal sinus abnormalities and the presence of extravascular eosinophils on a biopsy specimen.

The classical series of events in the evolution of CSS involves an initial phase characterized by asthma, often with rhinitis. In the second phase eosinophilic infiltration of tissues produces a variety of clinical disorders, including a pneumonia-like illness. Finally, a vasculitis develops that may involve any organ. The triphasic nature of CSS often leads to diagnostic difficulty since the clinicopathological findings change according to the stage of the disease. As in our case, the early presentation with adult-onset asthma and rhinitis is easily overlooked and the diagnosis only becomes apparent when a vasculitis develops.

Cutaneous lesions are commonly encountered in CSS, and since the skin serves as an accessible source of biopsy material the diagnosis can be made by a dermatologist. The main types of skin lesions found in CSS include erythematous macules and papules, urticarial weals, tender subcutaneous nodules with a predilection for the scalp and, as in our case, extensive purpura associated with necrosis and ulceration. The three main histological features are: (1) a necrotizing small-to-medium vessel vasculitis, (2) tissue infiltration by eosinophils and (3) extravascular granulomas. The diagnosis is strengthened by the presence of anti-myeloperoxidase antibodies (pANCA), which occur in approximately 50% of cases, and migratory pulmonary infiltrates on chest radiograph. Other extrapulmonary, extracutaneous manifestations of CSS include weight loss, mononeuritis multiplex, renal disease, cardiac disease and gastrointestinal tract involvement.

Most patients with CSS respond rapidly to systemic corticosteroids, although some require adjunctive immunosuppressive therapy with agents such as cyclophosphamide or azathioprine. Occasionally, as in our case, CSS may run a fulminant course that is resistant to aggressive immunosuppressive therapy and is ultimately fatal.

Learning points

1. Although the clinical features in this case were suggestive of meningococcal septicaemia, a skin biopsy demonstrated eosinophilic vasculitis, which led to the correct diagnosis of Churg–Strauss syndrome (CSS).
2. CSS should be considered in a patient who presents with a vasculitic rash and who has a circulating eosinophilia and a history of asthma and rhinitis.
3. The cutaneous manifestations of CSS include a maculopapular eruption, palpable purpura, urticaria, tender subcutaneous nodules and widespread cutaneous necrosis.

Reference

Diri E, Buscemi DM, Nugent KM. Churg–Strauss syndrome: diagnostic difficulties and pathogenesis. *Am J Med Sci* 2003; 352: 101–5.

See also case numbers 15, 40.

Index

T - #0519 - 071024 - C228 - 254/190/11 - PB - 9780367393441 - Gloss Lamination